Looking Within

The publisher gratefully

acknowledges the generous

contribution to this book

provided by the General

Endowment Fund of

the Associates of the

University of California Press

Looking Within

How X-Ray, CT, MRI, Ultrasound,
and Other Medical Images Are Created,
and How They Help Physicians Save Lives

ANTHONY BRINTON WOLBARST

Illustrations by Gordon Cook

UNIVERSITY OF CALIFORNIA PRESS

Berkeley   Los Angeles   London

University of California Press
Berkeley and Los Angeles, California

University of California Press, Ltd.
London, England

© 1999 by the Regents of the University of California

Library of Congress Cataloging-in-Publication Data
Wolbarst, Anthony B.
    Looking within : how X-Ray, CT, MRI, ultrasound, and other medical images
are created, and how they help physicians save lives / Anthony Brinton Wolbarst.
        p.   cm.
    Includes bibliographic references and index.
    ISBN 0-520-21181-2 (alk. paper) — ISBN 0-520-21182-0 (pbk. : alk. paper)
    1. Diagnostic imaging—popular works.   I. Title.
    RC78.7.D53W649   1999
    616.07'54—dc 21   98-3892

Drawings are by Gordon Cook.

Printed in the United States of America
9   8   7   6   5   4   3   2   1

The paper used in this publication meets the minimum requirements of American National Standards for
Information Sciences—Permanence of Paper for Printed Library Materials, ANSI Z39.48-1984.

For Eleanor

"She openeth her mouth with wisdom;
and in her tongue is the law of kindness"

Proverbs 31

Contents

Acknowledgments

Many people have helped me with this undertaking, and I am extremely grateful for the time and thought they contributed to it. They fall into three general groups: physicians, medical physicists, and family and friends not professionally involved with medicine.

Gregory Curt, clinical director of the National Cancer Institute, led me in the construction of about half of the patient case studies. Thanks, Greg, it was fun, and it was great to hear it from such a wonderful guide.

Three radiologists, John Chotkowski, Will McCann, and Dennis Patton, and especially an internist, Kevin Nealon, read the whole manuscript carefully and provided valuable input. Bruce Bowen and Mohsen Gharib, also radiologists, kindly gave me the clinical images and the interpretations of them that I used in putting together several of the case studies.

Robert Zamenhof, a medical physicist who taught me much of what I know of the physics of imaging, scrutinized all of *Looking Within*—twice—with his usual insight and good humor, and offered many ideas for improvements. Seong K. Mun and Allan Richardson also gave it a careful reading, and my thesis advisor, Bill Doyle, commented on the parts on MRI. Steve Bacharach provided a very helpful update on clinical PET; Allan Cormack on several occasions talked with me about the early days of CT; and Bill Hendee made sensible (as always) suggestions concerning my speculations on the future of imaging in chapter 9.

Several family members and other good friends who are not medically inclined were willing to be volunteered to read the manuscript from the point of view of nonmedical people. They found many areas that needed simplification or more lucid explanation, and their observations helped me eliminate a number of stumbling blocks. My thanks to Pete Detgen, Jay Hardgrove, Peter Head, Tom Fisher, Joe Mazzetti, and especially to my beautiful and clever country cousin, Ramsey Ludlow Sharratt, who said, at all the right places, "I'm just not sure this is completely clear."

I ran into Dana (Hastings) Murphy on the Metro, and she's just as sharp and funny as when she was a freshman at Smith, those few years ago. Dana agreed to do some sanding and polishing and, as a result, *Looking Within* is a good deal more readable than before she got to it. My copy editor at the University of California Press, Madeleine Adams, also did a splendid job in that regard.

Two people helped to turn what sometimes felt like two years at hard labor into a pleasure. My editor at the University of California Press, Howard Boyer, is a wise and supportive counselor, and has become a good friend. So also Gordon Cook, a gentle and amusing guy who is a delight to work with, and whose drawings (both here and in my *Physics of Radiology*) are nothing short of superb.

A number of physicians and other medical professionals took time from their busy schedules to respond to my requests for photographs. I have acknowledged them in the figure captions but I also want to give them my deep thanks here. In selecting photographs from among those sent by equipment manufacturers, I have attempted to achieve a fair and representative balance—weighted somewhat, I admit, by the degree to which they made serious efforts to provide images appropriate for a book such as this. But most important, I have chosen the photos that I feel most clearly illustrate the point. In no case should the use of a photograph be interpreted as an endorsement of a product.

I have tried hard to ensure the accuracy of what I have written, but I may have let some errors creep in. Or, as we say in Washington, mistakes may have been made. I would appreciate hearing from readers who find any.

Finally, I offer my deepest appreciation and my love to Eleanor Nealon, my bride of a dozen years. She is one tough literary critic, the coauthor of my dreams, and the loveliest lady I know. Eleanor, thank you for sharing your life with me.

Preface

A century ago, a doctor had no way to view the inside of a patient's body other than to cut it open.

That changed literally overnight on the evening of November 8, 1895, when Wilhelm Conrad Roentgen happened upon X rays. His extraordinary and mysterious radiation immediately covered the front pages of newspapers everywhere, and within months physicians throughout the world were using the pictures it produced to set broken bones and remove bullets. Roentgen had found "a new kind of rays," as he called them—and in so doing, he had discovered a splendid window for looking within the body and painlessly examining the organs and bones.

Medical imaging evolved steadily but slowly from then until the 1970s as researchers continually devised better ways to provide clinical information. The developments over the past few decades, by contrast, have been nothing short of revolutionary. Made possible and driven largely by the availability of powerful and inexpensive computers, computed tomography (CT) and then magnetic resonance imaging (MRI) have radically altered patient treatment and, beyond that, even the ways in which physicians perceive and think about the body.

American health care providers now perform over a quarter billion imaging examinations annually—one a year for every man, woman, and child, on average—and the curious among us would naturally like to know how those studies are made and what they are doing for and to us. *Looking Within* is intended to explain how X-ray, mammography, CT, MRI, nuclear medicine, ultrasound, and other medical images are created and used by physicians in caring for our families and ourselves. It describes, in nonspecialized but technically correct language, the remarkable technologies that enable doctors to visualize the organs and other tissues of the living body without having to slice them apart, and the essential roles that the resulting medical images play in the diagnosis and treatment of patients. You may be surprised by how easily all of them, even the more subtle ones like CT and MRI, can be grasped in simple yet realistic terms. The topic is inherently understandable and fascinating—especially so when our health is involved, or that of a loved one.

Every chapter beyond the first focuses on a specific kind of diagnostic imaging, providing a brief overview of how it works and what it can tell the clinician. Subsequent sections may delve more deeply into the most interesting aspects of the imaging technology and its operation. For imaging that requires a computer, as with CT and MRI, I include an elementary explanation of what it computes, and why. Where there are concerns about possible hazards, I discuss some of the recent evidence on the risks.

Each chapter also presents several patient cases that show how physicians employ images, combined with other information, in patient care. We shall explore the symptoms of a familiar medical problem; the image-derived information that is needed; the relevant imaging study, including the patient's experience of it; the physician's use of the image in diagnosis; the treatment; and the outcome and follow-up. While some of the situations sketched are medically not serious, such as a broken bone or a normal pregnancy, others involve life-threatening problems, like AIDS-related pneumonia, a heart attack, or breast cancer. Most people have had very little exposure to the thought processes of real physicians handling real cases—medical television programs, from *Dr. Kildare* on, have almost always centered on interpersonal issues, with a heavy peppering of medical jargon that may be all but meaningless to the viewer. In the cases presented here, the reader can follow the progress of simplified but authentic medical problems and experience first-hand the sorts of clinical decisions that physicians must make in arriving at a diagnosis and in planning the treatment.

In the current environment of managed care, moreover, it is helpful to have some knowledge of the commonly used medical technologies that affect us. Physicians and patients are increasingly called upon to justify studies involving expensive diagnostic tools. Given this emphasis on cost-effectiveness, old questions gain new importance: Which imaging modality is most sensitive and specific for a given or suspected medical condition? What kinds of information can mammography, or ultrasound, or MRI provide concerning, say, a lump in the breast? To what extent do their capabilities overlap, or do they tell us quite different things? It might be possible to obtain more of the relevant clinical data, albeit at significantly greater cost, with one of these technologies rather than another—but would it actually make a difference in patient care? This book should help the reader understand these difficult but critical questions, and then address them in a more informed manner.

Looking Within may also be of interest to medical professionals. Nearly all physicians—family practitioners, internists, pediatricians, surgeons, gynecologists, oncologists—are asked to interpret diagnostic images for patients, and sometimes to say something about the complex technologies behind them, too. This is true also for nurses and other medical staff. *Looking Within* can provide health care professionals with brief, ready-for-use explanations of the concepts that underlie the imaging technologies—how they function and what their strengths and weaknesses are—that can help them in educating their students and supporting their patients.

Medical imaging is an essential branch of modern medicine that combines dazzling, cutting-edge technologies with clinical applications that frequently spell the difference between life and death for patients. I hope that you will find this brief description of it informative, interesting, and useful—and perhaps even a first step toward your further exploration of this exciting and vitally important field.

A CAVEAT

Looking Within is definitely *not* a health care guidebook for treating yourself or anyone else. It explains, rather, how several very interesting and important medical technologies work, and it offers examples of their clinical applications. The book may help you to discuss aspects of a medical situation or examination with your physicians, but it must not be considered medical advice—that should come only from them.

As Albert Einstein is supposed to have said, "An explanation should be made as simple as possible, but no simpler." My patient cases are based on real medical problems, but I have removed some (or a lot) of the complexity from nearly all of them; retaining more detail would have complicated the stories without offering much insight for the reader. I have also streamlined the discussions of some physical and technical processes. I have often had to balance simplicity and directness of description against completeness and precision. To get the essential points across most clearly here, I have consistently favored the former, as long as the presentation could still remain fundamentally correct. A physicist or physician will know that things are actually more subtle than some of my statements might indicate—but I try always to stick close enough to reality so as not to be misleading. For anyone who wishes to dig a bit deeper, I suggest taking a look at my *Physics of Radiology*.

I

From the Watching of Shadows

"Our science is from the watching of shadows."
Ezra Pound, Canto 85

One hundred years ago, the German physicist Wilhelm Conrad Roentgen (figure 1) happened upon X rays. Although no one realized it at the time, this most extraordinary and mysterious discovery foreshadowed the quantum upheavals that would turn the physical sciences upside down in the early decades of the twentieth century. More immediately and spectacularly, though, it flung open a door that led into a new and completely unanticipated dimension in the practice of medicine—the ability to look within a patient's body without having to slice it open.

"A NEW KIND OF RAY"

It is difficult, from today's vantage point, to imagine just how primitive medicine actually was a century or so ago. The idea of surgery can still make anyone a little nervous, but in earlier days, it elicited feelings of sheer horror. Many are the stories of the wounded or seriously ill who begged for a hard blow to the head, or even death itself, rather than the ordeal of the knife. Alcohol and opium could induce some degree of numbness, but anesthetics—the kind that really knock you out, like ether and chloroform—were not in wide use before the American Civil War. The painkilling properties of nitrous oxide gas and ether had been known since around 1800, but deep anesthesia was not used in surgery until midcentury.

In those days, moreover, something like half of all patients who did en-

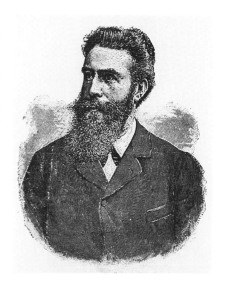

Figure 1. An engraving of Wilhelm Conrad Roentgen, published in 1896, less than a year after his discovery. From E. Trevert, *Something about X-Rays for Everyone* (1896; reprint, Madison, Wis.: Medical Physics Publishing Company, 1988). Shortly after this engraving was published, one visitor described Roentgen as "a very tall man, with a scholarly stoop, his face somewhat pockmarked, stern but kindly, and very modest in his remarks upon his achievements." Quoted in R. E. Mould, *A Century of X-Rays and Radioactivity in Medicine* (London: Institute of Physics Publishing, 1993), 2.

dure the amputation of an arm or leg died of infection anyway. It wasn't until the 1860s that Louis Pasteur, Joseph Lister, Florence Nightingale, and others recognized and began preaching the importance of cleanliness, disinfectants, and sterilized surgical instruments. But even with these improvements in the operating room (which, like anesthesia, took decades to gain general acceptance), death from infection was commonplace until penicillin and other antibiotics became readily available after World War II.

Medical diagnosis, too, was almost entirely art, and little science. The physician could measure body temperature, blood pressure, pulse rate, and a few simple chemical attributes of blood and urine, but not much else. Odors and subtle aspects of a patient's appearance commonly provided equally important clues. But a doctor often had no way to know what was going on within the body other than to cut it open.

All of that changed overnight in 1895. Roentgen, a respectable but rather obscure professor at the University of Würzburg, had been experimenting with an apparatus of widespread scientific interest at the time, a vacuum tube through which electric charges were flowing. Late in the evening of November 8, working in a darkened room, something unusual caught his eye: when an electric discharge occurred in his tube, a nearby piece of paper coated with a chemical compound of barium, platinum, and cyanide produced a glow. With his glass tube completely enveloped in black cardboard, no light from it could be reaching the coated paper. So something invisible had to be passing through the cardboard and reaching the barium platinum cyanide, inducing it to give off light. Roentgen had, in fact, discovered X-ray radiation by observing X-ray fluorescence

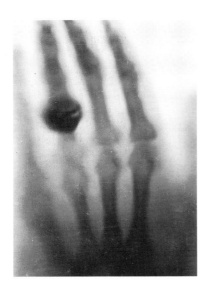

Figure 2. The earliest extant X-ray record, taken by Roentgen on December 22, 1895, of his wife's hand and signet ring. Courtesy of the Deutsches Roentgen-Museum, Remscheid-Lennep, Germany.

(the emission of light caused by an X-ray stimulus) in a nearby fluorescent material.

By placing various objects between the tube and his fluorescent screen, Roentgen learned that they affected the brightness of the emitted light by different amounts. Paper and cardboard had little effect, but a thick sheet of metal quenched the light completely. And when he held his hand in the path of the X-ray beam, he could make out the bones of his fingers projected in silhouette upon the screen. A short while later, Roentgen produced the first X-ray record, capturing for all time his wife's hand and signet ring on a glass photographic plate (figure 2).

Word of this wonder spread like wildfire, and the experiment was easy to reproduce. Within months, physicians throughout the world were using X-ray images to extract shrapnel and set broken bones. Roentgen had discovered "a new kind of ray," as he described them, and in so doing he had created a splendid window for looking within the living body.

For the better part of a century thereafter, innovations in the field of medical imaging came slowly but steadily, and a few were quite remarkable. But the advances in recent years have been as revolutionary as the computers that have made them possible. If the people who developed the automobile, the airplane, the telephone, or the television were to run across modern versions of their inventions, they would probably understand a great deal of what they found. But if Roentgen were to wander through a medical imaging center today, with its computed tomography (CT) scans, magnetic resonance imaging (MRI), and positron emission tomography (PET), much of what he saw would mystify him.

Looking Within will walk Herr Professor Roentgen, and anyone else who would like to come along, through a modern imaging department, explaining the medical marvels that would so amaze him. But let's start with a technology Roentgen should feel quite comfortable with, and show how an ordinary X-ray film study of a hand is produced and used today.

X - R A Y   F I L M   O F   A   C R A C K E D   B O N E

When a patient shows up at her door, a physician will listen to the symptoms, do a physical examination, and perhaps take some blood or urine specimens (which today can provide highly specific and valuable information). From her interpretation of the results, she can probably limit the diagnosis to one or a few possibilities. Medical imaging may now step in to play a decisive role in confirming, refining, modifying, or refuting the initial diagnosis. Imaging may also be invaluable in planning the treatment and in following the patient's progress over time.

It may not be readily apparent to the patient, but this general process of gathering relevant information on the malady, considering the possible explanations, and focusing first on the most likely ones goes on quietly even with as simple a problem as a broken bone.

Kathleen Nealon, the sixteen-year-old star pitcher for her high school softball team, took a hard blow to the left hand from a batted ball, causing a great deal of pain and rapid swelling. Her older sister, Kelly, who had dropped by to watch part of the game, drove her to the emergency room of the local hospital.

After carefully inspecting the hand, the emergency room physician sent Kathleen to the radiology department for an X-ray film. An imaging study was needed for a correct diagnosis that would, in turn, guide Kathleen's treatment. If no bones were damaged, Kathleen could get by with elevation of her hand, intermittent application of a cold pack, and medication to reduce swelling and discomfort. If the radiologist found a hairline crack, the hand might need a cast to counteract any stresses on the injury during healing. If a bone had been broken into separate pieces, it might even be necessary to wire them together surgically for proper setting. Before there were X-ray films, a physician would have had to stabilize a bone without being able to see clearly how to position the pieces, and that could result in weakness and deformity after mending.

Kathleen's X ray took less than five minutes. The radiographer (also known as a radiologic technologist) positioned her swollen hand on a *cassette*, which contained a sheet of radiographic film, adjusted the height of the X-ray tube above it, and reduced the dimensions of the rectangular X-ray beam until it barely covered the hand (figure 3a). Then he protected

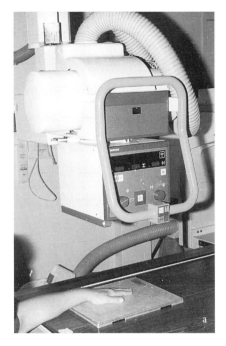
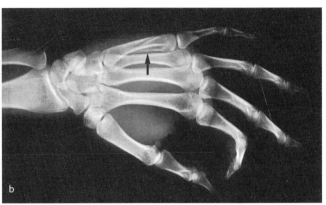

Figure 3. X-ray study of a hand. (a) A modern X-ray unit, with the X-ray tube (within the horizontal, white cylindrical housing) pointing its beam downward at the hand, which is resting on a film cassette. The corrugated hose carries the high voltage cables from the generator, which is outside the room, and tubes for circulating the coolant oil. The two knobs on the collimator assembly allow adjustment of the beam size, to minimize the amount of tissue irradiated. (b) In this film of the left hand, the arrow points to a clean break in the fifth metacarpal bone. Compare it with the normal fourth metacarpal, below.

Kathleen's body and neck with a lead-lined apron, which strongly absorbs any stray X rays. He stepped behind a shielding wall, set the controls of the X-ray machine, and kept watch on his patient through a lead-glass window as he shot the film. He then replaced the exposed film in the cassette with a fresh one, repositioned the hand, and took a second film.

In a few minutes, the films were developed and ready for inspection (figure 3b). Both were of high enough quality for the radiologist to identify the problem and guide Kathleen's treatment. As with most radiographic studies, the contrast between bone and soft tissue was high. There was almost no visual noise interfering with what had to be seen. And the films had sufficient sharpness and resolution of detail to reveal a clean, simple break in one of the bones into two separate pieces. These had not been displaced relative to one another, but the radiologist recommended a cast anyway, to ensure that the bone would be rigidly immobilized.

A month later, when the bone was nearly healed, the cast came off. A few weeks after that, Kathleen was back in there pitching.

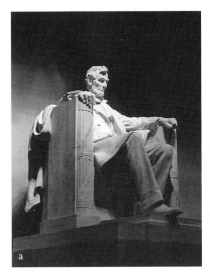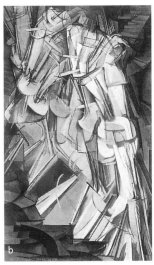

Figure 4. Images conveying different types of visual information. (a) The statue within the Lincoln Memorial is a highly realistic representation. Photo by Gordon Cook. (b) *Nude Descending a Staircase, No. 2* (1912), by Marcel Duchamp, abstractly depicts an essence of the human form by capturing its motion. Courtesy of the Philadelphia Museum of Art: Louise and Walter Arensberg Collection.

WHAT A PHYSICIAN NEEDS FROM A MEDICAL IMAGE

My wife and I live in Washington, and even though we visit the Lincoln Memorial with out-of-town friends two or three times a year, we never tire of it. We love it for the strength and integrity carved into the wonderfully lifelike face of the man, along with his gentle understanding and acceptance of human frailties (figure 4a). It's all right there, in the stone.

Another, and altogether different, visual treat is Marcel Duchamp's *Nude Descending a Staircase* (figure 4b). Duchamp interprets the human form by portraying its flow, and his painting is as abstract and impersonal a representation as *Lincoln* is solid and familiar.

Some would argue that *Lincoln* is a more important work, of greater inherent value because of its directness and traditional authenticity. No one ever has to ask what it means. Such a perspective would miss a crucial point: the two representations are intended to do very dissimilar things, and both succeed splendidly in their individual ways of depicting reality—but an informed interpretation is essential for a true appreciation of either.

The situation is much the same for a medical image. You might suppose that the value of a picture increases with its visual similarity to the part of the body that it examines. But much of that information content will invariably be medically irrelevant at best, or detract from or even hide the diagnostically critical features. Take a look at the studies by X ray, nuclear medicine, and magnetic resonance angiography (all of which we shall discuss later) in figure 5, and you'll see that what a physician has to work with can be quite distinct from photographic reality. What is important is

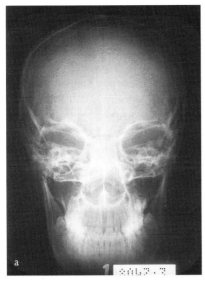

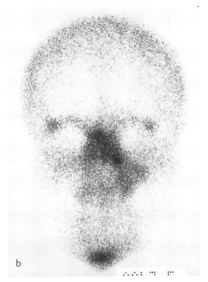

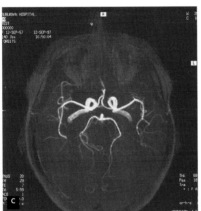

Figure 5. Three medical images of a head. (a) This radiograph illustrates the complexity of X-ray images in two dimensions, brought about by the overlapping of shadows from bone and other tissues. (b) A nuclear medicine scan can indicate portions of skull that take up too great, or too small, amounts of special, bone-seeking radioactive materials. (c) Magnetic resonance angiography images the arteries and veins by sensing faint changes in the magnetic properties of blood as it moves within applied magnetic fields that vary over time and space. Figures a and b courtesy of the American College of Radiology; figure c courtesy of Mohsen Gharib, Suburban Hospital, Bethesda, Md.

what he can "read" in the image. His job is to detect any significant anomaly in it, and identify a corresponding irregularity in the patient's body. He must then interpret this in terms of a deviation from normal anatomy or physiology—the what, how, and why of what has actually gone wrong with the cells, tissues, and organs. Only then, after settling on at least a tentative diagnosis, is it possible to choose the best treatment. A medical image will be considered good if it helps make any or all of this happen reliably and easily. A diagnostic imaging system must therefore be able to display the *specific*, distinctive aspects of a patient's anatomy or physiology that are causing a problem, and be *sensitive* enough to pick up even very faint signs of it.

The specificity, sensitivity, and other characteristics of the various imaging tools, in turn, are determined by how they work—and they work in remarkably disparate ways. But although the several imaging technologies use quite different physical processes in carrying out their appointed tasks, as we shall see, they do share a fundamental commonality of approach: they create medical images by following and recording, by some means, the progress of suitable probes that are attempting to pass through a patient's body. The body must be partially, but only partially, transparent to the probes. If the probes all slip right through bones and organs without interacting with them, like light through a pane of clear glass, no differences among the tissues can be visualized. Similarly, if their passage is completely blocked, nothing much shows up. But if we choose probes that are only somewhat absorbed, scattered, reflected, delayed, or otherwise affected, we may be able to detect small differences in how they interact with different biological materials. And these differences can then serve as the raw material for the creation of diagnostically useful pictures.

When a uniform beam of X rays entered Frau Roentgen's or Kathleen Nealon's hand, for example, the bones and muscles *attenuated* it (i.e., removed energy from it, reducing its intensity) by different amounts, thereby casting a distinctive pattern of X-ray shadows in it. The no-longer-uniform beam that emerged from the hand then fell upon and exposed a photographic plate or film cassette. Finally, the X-ray shadow pattern was distilled into a permanent visual record when the photographic plate or film was developed.

Mammographic radiography, nuclear medicine, magnetic resonance imaging, and ultrasound use different physical probes in examining the body. These probes interact with the tissue immediately around them, and the nature of that interaction can be highly sensitive not only to the specific physical characteristics of the tissue, but also to the nature of the probe. It should be no surprise, then, that each imaging technology, with its own particular kind of probe, is suitable for the study of only certain kinds of medical problems. A fine crack in a small bone that would not show up at all with ultrasound imaging (which uses high-frequency sound waves) or with magnetic resonance imaging (magnetic fields and radio waves) may be fully visible in an ordinary X-ray film and perhaps in some kinds of nuclear medicine studies as well (gamma rays). Conversely, subtle differences among the various soft tissues of the abdomen that cannot be seen with the X rays of radiography or even CT may be easy to spot with ultrasound or MRI. Different probes, different interactions with the tissues, and different means of detecting the probes give rise to different images conveying different types of clinical information.

The gamma-ray probes used in nuclear medicine originate within the body, and are detected after they leave it, but the basic idea is much the same.

A test that is not specific, or selective, enough may light up and suggest a medical problem when, in fact, none exists; such a false positive result can cause the patient needless anxiety and lead to unneeded further tests, treatments, and costs. A false negative from an insufficiently sensitive measurement, on the other hand, may preclude the treatment of a condition that is actually serious. Unfortunately, no test can be perfectly specific and sensitive, so there always will be some incorrect readings.

Selecting the technology that employs the most appropriate probe is only the first step. Given that the physician chooses a suitable diagnostic test, the resulting pictures will be of little clinical use unless they are of good enough *image quality.* Although there are other critical factors as well, the three gold standards by which images (and the imaging systems that produce them) are most commonly judged are contrast, resolution, and visual noise.

When *contrast* is good, significant physical differences among the tissues show up as substantial differences in shades of gray (or color) in the image. The contrast between bone and the soft tissues of muscle or the internal organs, for example, is almost always strong in a radiograph, even in Roentgen's first plate—but there is little inherent radiographic contrast among the organs themselves, so it is sometimes difficult to see them at all. The same organs might show up with dazzling contrast, however, with an MRI or a nuclear medicine scan.

Some kinds of investigations, such as the search for calcifications in the breast (tiny flecks of bonelike material that may sometimes be suggestive of cancer), require high *resolution* (also called *sharpness*), the ability to display fine detail. X-ray films tend to provide extremely good resolution, and tiny objects and linelike features of interest within the body (such as the crack in Kathleen's finger, figure 3b) may show up well in a radiograph or mammogram. One important source of *un*sharpness is the blur introduced by patient movement—which is the reason for the inevitable "Take a deep breath and hold it!" that accompanies chest films. With some kinds of imaging, such as ultrasound and nuclear medicine, the power of resolution is inherently not great; but although those technologies may get low marks in visualizing anatomic detail, they do display the contrast needed to provide other (sometimes much more important) sorts of information on the patient's medical condition—such as how healthy the tissues of a particular organ are.

Visual noise refers to anything that interferes, a little or a lot, with an image, just as static noise from lightening in a storm will degrade a radio broadcast. An all-too-familiar example of visual noise (before the advent of cable) was the irritating snow that blew across your TV screen whenever the signal was too weak. But noise may assume more subtle forms, as anyone who has enjoyed an afternoon in the park with Georges Seurat well knows. His *Sunday on La Grande Jatte* is composed of countless little dabs of paint of various colors. From a distance, the image seems quite smooth and realistic (figure 6a), but the finer features are indistinguishable. At close range, the size of the individual dabs causes the picture to take on

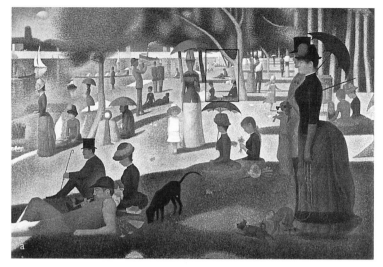
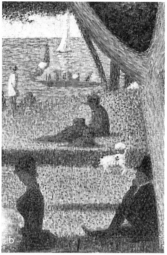

Figure 6. *A Sunday on La Grande Jatte,* by Georges Seurat. (a) The painting seems smooth-textured from a normal viewing distance. (b) Close inspection reveals a pointillistic pattern similar to the kind of visual noise that sometimes occurs in radiographs and other medical images. Courtesy of the Art Institute of Chicago, Helen Birch Bartlett Memorial Collection.

You can see another example of visual noise in the photographic reproductions of this book. The pointillistic printing technique causes a loss of visual information (or, equivalently, introduces a kind of visual noise), though it usually isn't distracting to the reader. Even with the original photographs, moreover, a microscope will show that what looks like a homogeneous dark gray area is actually an illusion produced by millions of closely spaced, but separate, microscopic flecks of silver metal.

a speckled texture (figure 6b), and that, too, limits the amount of sharpness possible. Fine detail is not what Seurat had in mind, but the objectives of medical imaging are different. A digital image, for example, is composed of a hundred thousand or more tiny dots of different shades of gray or color, and the imaging system must be designed to ensure that they are small and numerous enough for a picture to be clinically useful—otherwise, it may appear blotchy, too noisy to be of value.

We have been discussing the factors that underlie the selection of a technology with sufficient specificity and sensitivity for a given job, and the need for its images to be of adequate quality. Figure 7a, a candid portrait of young Nadine Wolbarst, nicely illustrates these ideas. So as not to produce just one more cute-kitten photo, I worked diligently to reveal the essence of her character by capturing, specifically, her glazed-over, catnip-deranged stare. The imaging equipment had to be sensitive enough, moreover, to perform in the challenging environment of a dimly lit suburban Washington den. Fortunately, disposable-camera film technology (with flash) was up to the demands, and the results exceeded my wildest artistic aspirations.

Figure 7b shows how the photo was made: Nadine was bathed in light, some of which was reflected toward the camera. The lens projected the pattern of light coming from her onto the film. The more light that struck a tiny area of film, the darker it would become when it was chemically de-

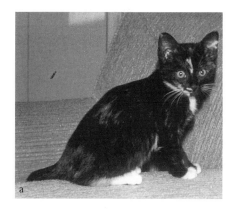

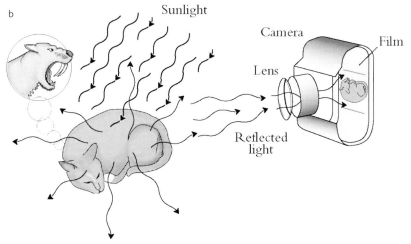

Figure 7. Contrast, resolution, and noise level are three important qualities that affect the ability of any image to convey information. (a) Nadine Wolbarst appears with high contrast, sharp resolution, and little visual noise. (b) The making of a photograph: light reflecting from a spot on Nadine's coat is focused onto a corresponding point on the film within the camera.

Sunlight

Camera

Film

Lens

Reflected light

veloped later; thus, the camera produced a "negative." The process was then repeated, in effect, but this time with the negative (rather than Nadine herself) serving as the source of the incoming pattern of light; the negative from this negative was the "positive" shown in figure 7a.

Technically speaking, figure 7a is not a bad picture. There is good contrast, easily picking up the shades of gray in Nadine's coat. The resolution is fine enough for us to make out her whiskers, and there is virtually no visual noise. Most important, at least with respect to the storage and transfer of information, the specificity, sensitivity, and overall visual quality are sufficient for you or me, the final link in the imaging chain, to determine that this is indeed a cat. And I, with access to certain additional data, can even assert with a fair degree of assurance which cat she usually is. If the film were underexposed or blurry, or in some other sense carried less information or more noise, then that would not necessarily be true.

Turning these thoughts back to medicine: no single technology can perform all imaging tasks well, so a physician must understand what the different types of medical images can reveal about a patient's condition.

Only then can he or she choose the technology most likely to provide the essential, specific piece of information needed to address a given medical problem. Then it's up to the medical imaging staff to produce pictures of high enough quality to allow a reliable interpretation and diagnosis. And all of this has to be done with minimal risk to the patient and staff, and at an acceptable cost.

WHAT IMAGING STUDIES REVEAL

Six general kinds of imaging are used routinely in modern diagnostic clinics: radiography, fluoroscopy (including studies that involve the computer), computed tomography, nuclear medicine, magnetic resonance imaging, and ultrasonography. The most familiar of these, of course, is radiography, the taking of X-ray films.

Radiography

As indicated above, medical images are generally produced by tracking the progress of suitable probes as they pass through the body. A beam of X rays consists of such probes (figure 8a). Think of an X-ray beam as a stream made up of vast numbers of small, discrete, particlelike bundles of energy, called photons. (Appendix A provides an elementary review of atoms and radiation.) X-ray photons propagate through space in straight lines and at the speed of light. Most important, they can collide with atoms and in this way be removed from the beam. In conventional radiography, a uniform, penetrating beam produced by an X-ray tube exposes a part of the body for a fraction of a second (figure 8b). Since the various tissues reduce the intensity of different areas of the beam by different amounts, an X-ray shadow is imprinted in the beam before it exits the patient. The shadow pattern that emerges is then captured on special photographic film. The more a bone or other tissue in the beam path absorbs or scatters X rays, the smaller the number of them that make it completely through to expose the film—and the clearer (less dark) the corresponding region of film will appear after it is developed.

X-ray films are most useful in locating and examining objects that have densities significantly greater or less than the surrounding soft tissues—as with bullets, bones, or lungs. X rays are also excellent for examining veins and arteries or parts of the gut if these areas can be filled with "contrast agent," such as certain compounds of iodine or barium, which soak up X rays particularly well. A tumor, unfortunately, presents more of a challenge. Because its density may be close to that of the surrounding healthy organ and muscle tissues, a cancer growth may give rise to little radiographic contrast, and so may be difficult (or impossible) to see di-

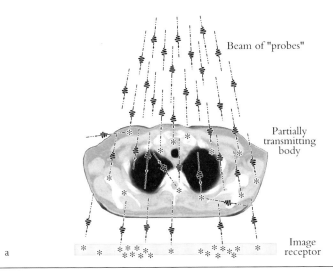

Beam of "probes"

Partially
transmitting
body

Image
receptor

a

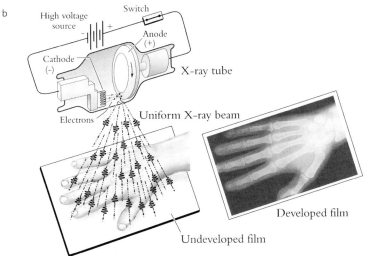

b

Switch

High voltage
source

Anode
(+)

Cathode
(-)

X-ray tube

Electrons

Uniform X-ray beam

Developed film

Undeveloped film

Figure 8. Standard X-ray filming, or radiography. (a) An X-ray image of a part of the body can be produced by keeping track of the fate of "probes" that enter it and do, or do not, interact with it. (b) Overview of the radiographic process. During the fraction of a second that the exposure switch is closed, so that high voltage from the generator is briefly being applied to the X-ray tube, the tube creates a nearly uniform X-ray beam, which enters a part of the body. Only some X-ray photons pass through; the rest are scattered or absorbed, predominantly in the denser tissues, especially the bones. The patterns imprinted in the (no longer uniform) residual X-ray beam emerging from the far side of the patient are captured on specialized photographic film in a cassette. Where more radiation passes through the patient and reaches the cassette, the developed film will be darker.

rectly on an X-ray film. Yet a tumor may reveal its presence by altering the appearance of an adjacent body (such as the wall of bowel that contains contrast agent) that *can* be visualized.

The inherently very high resolution of X-ray films enables them to provide critical details of fine structure, revealing hairline cracks in bone, for instance, and irregularities in narrow blood vessels enhanced with contrast agent.

Finally, it's easy to control most visual noise in film radiography, and it rarely causes difficulties, unless the film is under- or overexposed.

Conventional X-ray radiography is still the most common and least expensive way of obtaining diagnostic medical and dental images, and for many tasks it is perfectly adequate. But imaging departments have other options to choose from, as well, and in many situations one or more of them may offer a far better approach to a clinical problem.

Fluoroscopy

Fluoroscopy is radiography's first cousin. Here, the X rays that pass through and emerge from the patient do not immediately expose a film. Instead, they are projected onto the front face of an image intensifier (figure 9), an electronic vacuum-tube device that transforms a life-size pattern of X-ray shadows into a small, bright optical image. This visible image can be fed into a film camera; more commonly, it goes to a television (video) camera, where it is converted into an electrical signal and sent to a video

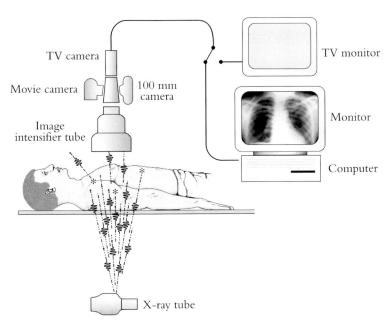

Figure 9. Fluoroscopy. The radiant energy from an X-ray tube passes through the patient, and the resulting X-ray shadows are transformed by the image intensifier into a bright image of visible light three centimeters or so in dimensions. This optical image, in turn, is captured by a 100 mm camera, a movie camera, or a video camera.

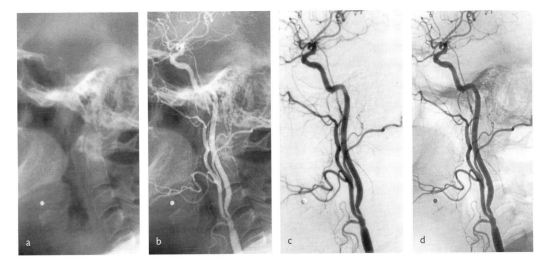

Figure 10. Digital subtraction angiography. For this DSA image of a carotid artery of the neck, a narrow catheter is threaded into a leg artery, up the aorta, and into the carotid. Images are obtained both (a) before, and (b) after a bolus of iodine-based contrast agent is injected through the tip of the catheter. (c) Aligning the two pictures and subtracting the "before" image from the "after," point by point, yields a "difference" image that shows only the vessels just filled with the iodine. (d) It may help with interpretation to reintroduce some faint background landmarking.

monitor for live display. The image can be recorded on videotape for subsequent playback and further processing.

As with X-ray filming, fluoroscopy is most adept at distinguishing objects that differ significantly from soft tissue in density. Its major advantage is that it lets a physician watch bodily processes in "real time," as they happen—for example, the movement of barium contrast agent (given orally or by enema) past partial obstructions in the gut, or the passage of injected iodine-based compounds through constrictions in blood vessels.

By itself, fluoroscopy finds many routine applications in the clinic, but its considerable powers are extended even further when it is coupled to a computer. Digital subtraction angiography (DSA), in particular, is splendid for imaging arteries and veins—nothing else shows up on the screen *but* the arteries and veins (figure 10). The computer stores separate fluoroscopic images before and after contrast agent is injected into the patient's bloodstream. It then subtracts the first image from the second, point by point, and displays the difference between the two as a new image. This third, "difference" image highlights those (and only those) places where the first and second images differ, that is, where blood vessels hold contrast agent; all the uninteresting, and easily confusing, background patterns are eliminated.

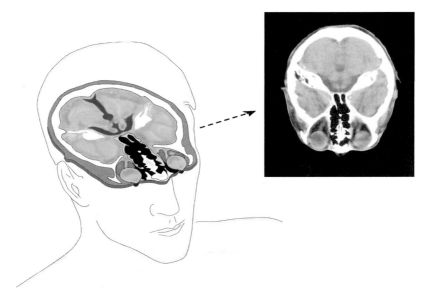

Figure 11. Computed tomography. This view of a slice of bone, eyes, and brain tissues several millimeters thick displays good soft-tissue contrast and detail, and low visual noise.

Computed Tomography (CT)

Conventional radiographic and fluoroscopic images are relatively straight-forward and inexpensive to produce—even the smallest X-ray clinics have the equipment—and the trained eye can often derive more than enough from them for an accurate diagnosis. But the superimposed shadows from overlapping tissues sometimes obscure the critical details that a physician needs to see.

What is captured by film or fluoroscopy, and is thereby available for diagnosis, is the pattern of X rays transmitted through the body. The radiographic process is thus a kind of condensation, or deflation, of patient anatomy from the real world of three dimensions into a visual image in two. In the process, the shadows from an intricate three-dimensional structure, like a head, can be flattened into hopeless chaos on film, as in figure 5a. Although a radiologist may be able to perform near magic in detecting and interpreting slight irregularities amidst all the junk, in many cases there is simply too much visual confusion.

Digital subtraction angiography provides one path around that problem, but it works only for blood vessels. Computed tomography achieves the same end for a wide variety of organs, but it produces images quite differently. CT (called "see-tee" or "cat scanning") uses X rays, an elaborate radiation detection system, and a computer that carries out millions of calculations to construct the image of a thin, breadlike (transverse) slice

LOOKING WITHIN

of the patient's body (figure 11). By eliminating the interfering patterns that come from over- and underlying bones and organs, CT provides ample contrast among the various soft tissues, far better than standard radiography or fluoroscopy can do. So CT is routinely used for detailed studies of abdominal and pelvic organs, the lungs, and the brain. CT can image objects down to about 1/3 millimeter (one millimeter is roughly 1/25 inch); although that is not nearly as fine as the resolution in standard radiography, it is good enough for many diagnostic needs.

In the mid 1970s, CT gave physicians a whole new way of seeing, and the resulting effect on patient care has been incalculable. More recently, CT has had to face stiff competition from MRI, which provides clinical information that is usually comparable, and sometimes far superior. Still, when either modality can do a job just as well, the considerably lower costs of CT normally make it the appropriate choice.

Nuclear Medicine

Stolen cars and those bewildered wildebeests on *Wild Kingdom* can be located easily if they carry small radio transmitters. Nuclear medicine employs the same principle.

A nuclear medicine study makes use of a radioactive chemical substance, called a radiopharmaceutical, that displays two essential characteristics: it concentrates within a particular site in the body, an organ or tissue of interest, and it emits gamma rays. It thereby becomes a localized transmitter of gamma radiation. Radioactive atoms of the element technetium, for example, can be attached to microscopic clumps of molecules of a certain protein. When injected into the bloodstream, these radioactively tagged chunks become temporarily stuck in the narrowest blood vessels of the lung. Then, just as a red-hot poker glows in a dark room, a lung containing the technetium-labeled clumps will "glow" gamma rays. The gamma rays coming from the lung can then be detected and processed by a gamma camera and made into an image, as in figure 12.

Gamma rays are inherently the same as X rays, but of different origin. They are emitted from the unstable nuclei of radioactive atoms, rather than created electronically in an X-ray tube. It is the source of the radiation, not the radiation itself, that distinguishes gamma-ray from X-ray photons.

A nuclear medicine image has relatively low spatial resolution; all you can see is the rough shape and size of the organ or tissue of interest. But if a part of the organ fails to take up the radioactive material, is missing, or is eclipsed by abnormal overlying tissues, then the corresponding region of the image will appear dark. Conversely, any part of the organ that takes up an excess of radiopharmaceutical will look unusually bright on the display. So a nuclear medicine image provides information principally on the physiology and pathology of an organ—what big parts of it are doing, or doing wrong—not the details of its anatomy.

Nuclear medicine began in the late 1930s when radioactive iodine was employed to investigate thyroid disease, and now it can contribute valu-

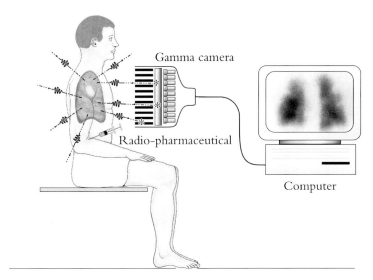

Gamma camera

Radio-pharmaceutical

Computer

Figure 12. Nuclear medicine. This examination of a patient's lungs reveals a region that has failed to take up a normal amount of radiopharmaceutical. The vessels leading to it may be blocked off by an obstruction, such as a blood clot, or perhaps normal lung tissue has been displaced by a tumor.

able information on nearly every organ. It has also worked well in the imaging of some tumors, providing an especially sensitive test of the spread of cancer from one organ to another. For cardiac patients, it furnishes quantitative assessments of the heart's capacity to pump blood.

One area where standard nuclear medicine has fallen largely out of favor (having been displaced by CT) is in brain imaging. Ironically, that's where positron emission tomography (PET) made its first important inroads. PET is a highly specialized form of nuclear medicine that utilizes a few unusual and difficult-to-produce atomic nuclei known as positron emitters in its radiopharmaceuticals, and some very complex and expensive imaging equipment. PET studies are particularly intriguing to neuroscientists and psychiatrists, since they can sometimes reveal the part of the brain where neural activity changes when certain mental processes are occurring. Figure 13a is a typical transverse-slice PET scan, at about the same level within the subject's head as figure 11, showing the distribution of water that has been labeled with a positron-emitting isotope of oxygen. One can stack many such slices to create a corresponding three-dimensional PET image. Figure 13b, for example, shows the differences that occur in such a three-dimensional map when a subject begins focusing on a specified task. The bright areas indicate *changes* in blood flow in the regions where the nerve cells are most active—in other words, not only is a new bunch of neurons starting to think deep thoughts, it is even managing to direct the circulatory system to divert extra jolts of fuel and oxygen there. To provide

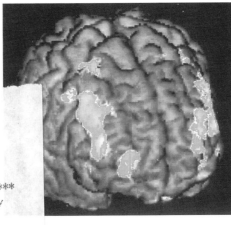

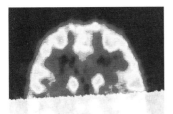
Transverse, CT-like slice of the
mages, one can construct a three-
"difference" image, mapping the
with changes in brain activity) that
emory task. To help with anatomic
uperimposed on a rendering of the
th magnetic resonance imaging. The
esy of Karen F. Berman, National

nce" image has been superimposed
ned separately with MRI.

_ PET difference-images for people
suffering from schizophrenia and other mental diseases look quite different from the normal. It may be difficult or impossible to explain what really causes such distinctions in terms of particular networks of nerve cells
and blood vessels, but the images may still be diagnostically useful. Fortunately, you don't always have to understand a medical phenomenon
completely to recognize it and deal with it effectively.

Long an important research tool in neurology, PET has recently been
finding clinical applications, too, such as in assessing the suitability of a
heart for bypass surgery and in searching for tumors.

Magnetic Resonance Imaging

Magnetic resonance imaging (MRI) not only reveals the structural details
of the various organs, as does CT, but it also provides information on their
physiological status and pathologies, as does nuclear medicine. And with
MRI, there is no radiation risk to the patient, since no X-ray or gamma-ray
energy is involved. Instead, MRI uses magnetic fields and radio waves to
probe the (nonradioactive) nuclei of hydrogen atoms occurring naturally
in the water molecules within and around cells.

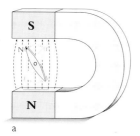

a

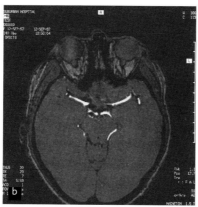

b

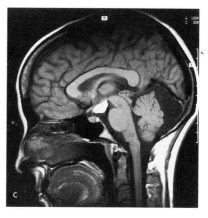

c

Figure 14. Magnetic resonance imaging. (a) The nuclei of the hydrogen atoms of water are magnetic, like tiny compass needles, and tend to align when placed in the field of a powerful magnet. When they are disturbed, they return to their equilibrium configuration by means of spin relaxation processes analogous to (though different from) that of a nudged compass needle. (b) This MRI image, taken at about the same level as figure 11, reveals subtle spatial variations in proton relaxation times, attributable to small differences in tissue type or physiologic status. (c) A side view of the head, which CT cannot produce with this degree of resolution. Figure b courtesy of Mohsen Gharib, Suburban Hospital, Bethesda, Md.

Imagine a compass needle (which itself is a tiny bar magnet) aligned comfortably along the Earth's magnetic field. Now, in your mind's eye, twist it through 180 degrees, so that it points south, and then release it. It will flop back over, oscillate a few times with diminishing swings, and eventually come to rest pointing north again (figure 14a). The amount of time this settling-down process takes is known as the *relaxation time*.

Somewhat similar processes can occur with the magnetic nuclei of atoms in the cells of your body in a strong magnetic field, and it is these that MRI uses for imaging. Here is the central concept underlying how magnetic resonance imaging works: MRI produces a map of variations in the relaxation times of the hydrogen nuclei in the water molecules of tissues. But those relaxation times depend on the types of tissues involved, and even on their state of health. So by sensing slight differences in proton relaxation in physiologically different tissues, MRI can generate an image that distinguishes among them.

This may require a little more explaining. The nucleus of a hydrogen atom is a single proton, which behaves in some ways like a tiny magnet. The positively charged proton seems to be spinning rapidly and, as with any other moving electrical charge (such as current in a wire), it creates its own small magnetic field, rather like that of the compass needle. You can think of the "needle" as pointing along the proton's axis of rotation. So when a patient lies in the magnetic field of an MRI device, many of the hydrogen nuclei of the water molecules in the tissues will end up with their spin axes lying parallel to the field.

It is then possible, by beaming in radio waves of the correct frequency, to make a few of these protons flip over and point in the opposite (i.e., the wrong) direction instead. Immediately, however, protons will begin to undergo a kind of spontaneous relaxation analogous to (but quite different from) that of our compass needle, in which they flop back into their more comfortable, normal alignment, with the spin axis lying back along the field. The average time it takes for a bunch of protons to return to their stable, equilibrium condition is called a *spin relaxation time*.

MRI creates images out of what are, in effect, measurements of spin relaxation times of hydrogen nuclei. That is, an MRI device maps out, point by point within a part of the body, variations in the proton relaxation times of the intracellular and other water within the tissues. There are two related, but distinct, clinically important spin relaxation processes that can occur in any tissue, with times called T_1 and T_2. These are sensitive to, and reflect, subtle aspects of the interactions of the water molecules with the various other molecules in the tissue; the characteristics of those other molecules, in turn, depend on the type and physiological status of the cells that contain them.

Images that emphasize spatial variations in T_1 or T_2 show how rapidly these two, somewhat different, relaxation processes take place everywhere in a slice or volume of tissue. And even where tissues seem exactly alike to X rays, so that CT offers no helpful information, one or both of these forms of MRI image may be able to distinguish clearly between different organs, and even between healthy and pathological forms of the same tissue type, with splendid clarity.

MRI works by way of physical processes totally unlike those of CT, but it produces pictures that are remarkably similar to CT scans (figure 14b). It displays a degree of contrast among soft tissues that is often much better than that of CT. And MRI images can reveal subtleties in the physiology of an organ, not just its anatomy. It can even provide high-resolution anatomic views that CT simply cannot generate, as with figure 14c. The only serious drawback of MRI is the high cost of acquisition and operation, though this is decreasing.

Ultrasound

Unlike the other imaging technologies we have discussed, ultrasonography does not involve electromagnetic radiation, such as gamma and X rays or light or radio waves. Ultrasound is a *mechanical* disturbance, rather, in which oscillations of 1 to 10 million hertz (Hz; cycles per second) travel

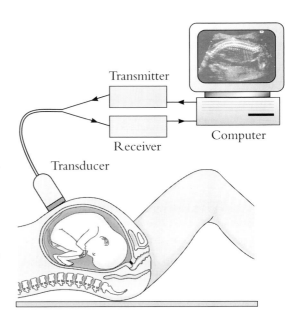

Figure 15. Ultrasound. A narrow beam of high-frequency sound directed into the patient is swept back and forth, and an image is created out of the echoes produced at the boundaries between different tissue. Although not comparable to that of a radiograph, the resolution of this ultrasound picture is fine enough to pick out the individual vertebral bodies and ribs of a fetus.

through soft tissues and fluids. (Humans with excellent ears typically can hear in the range 20 to 20,000 Hz.) In ultrasound imaging, a narrow beam of pulses of very high-frequency sound energy is directed into the body and swept back and forth; pictures of organs, blood vessels, and other structures are created out of the waves reflected back (figure 15).

When a pulse of ultrasound passes through different tissues, echoes are produced at the boundaries that contain or separate them. The *time* of return for each echo is proportional to the depth within the patient of the interface that produced it. The echo's intensity (*amplitude*) depends on that, and also on the differences in the acoustical characteristics of the materials on the two sides of the interface. A computer untangles all the data on echo times and intensities, and from that constructs images that can bring into view the beating of a heart or the stirring of an unborn child.

Since the probes in ultrasound are bundles of vibrations propagating through the body, image contrast among soft tissues depends primarily on differences in their *elastic* properties.

In many situations, ultrasound can provide critical clinical information quickly and inexpensively—for example, distinguishing a fluid-filled cyst from a solid tumor in the abdomen or the breast. It can assist in diagnosing a wide range of diseases, such as pathological changes in the liver, thyroid, gall bladder, pancreas, kidneys, heart, and the blood vessels. Ultrasound even serves as a guide in carrying out invasive procedures, such as draining an abscess. As with MRI, there is no X radiation involved, and it appears that a properly performed ultrasound study poses little risk to the patient. That is one reason it is used extensively to provide information about pregnancies—most importantly on certain fetal abnormalities—and as a visual aid in performing amniocentesis. Largely because of its cost-effectiveness and safety, some insurance companies and HMOs favor ultrasound for many kinds of examinations, and its role in the clinic will doubtless continue to expand.

Endoscopy

Finally, perhaps the simplest way to look within the body is, well, just to look. Physicians had long used rigid tubes, mirrors, and candles or sunlight to peer down the throat and along other bodily passageways, but it was the introduction of fiber optics in the 1950s that transformed the endoscope into a powerful modern clinical tool for direct clinical inspection.

Light entering the tip of a flexible glass fiber, a tenth of a millimeter or so across, will reflect again and again off its interior surface, like a stone skipping on water, and can travel great distances with little loss of intensity. A bundle of thousands of fibers, with lenses at the two ends, can carry a clear and sharp optical image. A modern endoscope consists of such a bundle, along with another bunch of fibers that bring in bright light to illuminate the region being viewed. In addition, it may have channels to convey gases or liquids in or out, or perhaps even a mechanical device, such as a biopsy forceps, at its business end. Endoscopy can be employed wherever there is an opening into the body, whether naturally occurring or surgical, and the equipment has become highly specialized for various applications.

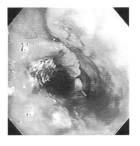

Figure 16. Endoscopic view of a tumor of the esophagus; a healthy esophagus looks like a smooth tube. Courtesy of Kevin Nealon, Chevy Chase, Md.

As will be apparent from the case studies in this book, endoscopy may pick up where other imaging techniques leave off. Fluoroscopy may indicate the presence of a tumor of the esophagus, for example, but an endoscope then obtains the biopsy needed for confirmation (figure 16). Likewise, after angiography reveals a partial blockage of a coronary artery, a high-power laser beam carried by a special fiber optic bundle of an endoscope may burn it away.

An area where endoscopy is receiving much attention is small-incision-hole surgery. The endoscope enters the body through a cut as little as one centimeter long, and it either brings in the necessary surgical instruments itself or guides their use. While such operations are much less traumatic to the patient and result in shorter hospital stays (both of which reduce cost), the procedures require additional training for the surgeon.

I hope these brief sketches of the principal imaging technologies have whetted your appetite for a deeper understanding of them. If you like to know at the outset of a book whodunit, or at least how it's done, you can sneak a peek at the table in the epilogue that summarizes the physical processes involved in creating the various kinds of images, and their respective strengths and weaknesses.

THE TRADEOFF:
BENEFITS VERSUS RISKS AND COSTS

X rays radically transformed the practice of medicine, but early on they revealed their dark side as well. Even before the turn of the century, researchers were reporting cases of horrible tissue burns caused by the radiation, some of which were fatal. Under the standard conditions used in diagnosis now, exposures high enough to cause such gross tissue damage are completely preventable. Unfortunately, though, radiation burns are not the only problem.

Laboratory experiments on cells and animals and epidemiological studies of exposed populations indicate that even at dose levels far below those that cause burns, X rays can nonetheless occasionally (but do not necessarily) induce cancers and birth defects. There is, however, a major problem with those midrange dose-response studies; the doses for which radiogenic (radiation-produced) cancers have actually been observed may be less than the burn level, but they are still a good deal higher than those that a patient receives in nearly any modern radiological examination. In other words, the midrange dose-effect study results can tell us almost nothing with assurance about the cancer risks at the very low-dose levels encountered in most X-ray or gamma-ray imaging. And direct evidence on the real risks from diagnostic amounts of radiation simply does not exist. Fortunately, what we do have suggests that the risks from today's diagnostic procedures are extremely small.

There is a fundamental tradeoff between the expected (but not certain) medical benefits and the highly unlikely (but possible) hazards from an X-ray examination; so also for other imaging methodologies. Over the years, medicine has learned to strike a proper balance between the recognized diagnostic advantages of imaging and the very small, but nevertheless real, possibility that serious, radiation-caused cancers and other adverse health effects might ensue from any study.

In the next chapter I shall say more about ways to gauge the risks for X rays. For now, I simply repeat that the estimated likelihood of someone becoming ill from a medically indicated, properly conducted diagnostic procedure is very, very small. The risk should be compared, moreover, with the probably far greater risk from *not* having the procedure performed, in which case a patient's treatment may be considerably less than optimal. So when someone asks, "Is this X-ray exam completely safe?" a good answer is usually: "We don't know for certain, but it's surely much safer than not doing the examination."

But what about the high costs of providing state of the art clinical care to large numbers of people? Hundreds of billions of dollars, a significant part of the gross domestic product, are spent each year on health care. A sizable block of this goes for the purchase and operation of big-ticket, high-tech medical equipment. Certainly, we all want the best possible diagnostic capabilities for those we love and for ourselves, but health care providers have to think carefully about whether one or another particular piece of costly apparatus is truly essential for proper treatment.

And as a community, we have but a finite pot of money. Given this limitation, would we all be significantly better off with a new MRI machine in the local hospital? Or with guardrails and lighting on that awful road that runs along the cliff, or with more police, or with better-paid teachers in the schools? Clearly, the benefits and the costs of imaging and other medical technologies must be weighed against the pros and cons of addressing our other major needs—and only through such an ongoing process can health care providers and society as a whole make intelligent decisions on the development and use of those technologies.

Fortunately, one of the most valuable forms of imaging, and certainly the most common, is also among the least expensive: ordinary X-ray filming. It is also the easiest to describe. So let us begin our full-fare tour of an imaging center with a visit to the X-ray suite.

CHAPTER 2

Shadows on X-Ray Film
RADIOGRAPHY / MAMMOGRAPHY

Archimedes conceived of a method for assessing the purity of precious metals, legend has it, in a flash of inspiration of heroic proportions. He leaped from his bath and raced naked through the streets of Syracuse shouting, "Eureka! Eureka!"—"I have found it! I have found it!" That isn't exactly what happened when Roentgen discovered X rays.

"ROENTGEN HAS SURELY GONE CRAZY"

Wilhelm Conrad Roentgen was born in the Rhineland in 1845, the only child of a Dutch mother and a wealthy German father, a textile merchant. Three years later, the family moved to Holland, where Wilhelm's early academic career was notable mainly for his expulsion from high school for disciplinary reasons—he refused to inform on a fellow student who had penned an unflattering caricature of one of the teachers. He attended the new Polytechnikum in Zurich, obtaining a diploma in mechanical engineering in 1868. He received his doctorate in physics from the highly regarded University of Zurich eleven months later, and then held academic positions in Würzburg, Strassburg, Hohenheim, Strassburg again, and Giessen.

The year 1895 found him back at the University of Würzburg as professor of physics and director of the Physics Institute. The position came with some substantial perks, including living quarters on the upper floor of the Institute and a well-stocked wine cellar. The author of forty-eight publications, Roentgen had achieved a solid reputation among physicists for his meticulous experiments on the elasticity of solids, the movement of liquids in narrow tubes, the conduction and absorption of heat by gases, and piezoelectricity (which, as we shall see later, plays an essential role in ultrasound imaging). Recently his interest had turned to cathode rays.

Voltage is often compared to water pressure, and electrical current to flow. Water flow through a segment of pipe that is partially plugged with a rag increases as the pressure at the entry side goes up; likewise, current through an electrical resistance is proportional to the applied voltage.

Scientists had long been intrigued by what happens when a high voltage is applied between two metal electrodes inside a partially evacuated glass vessel. The gas within would glow, investigators knew, as would the glass itself in the area near the anode (the electrode attached to the positive pole of the voltage source). It was assumed that the agent responsible for this phenomenon was some sort of particle or wave, perhaps negatively charged, that emerged from the cathode (the negative electrode) and flowed toward the anode. These so-called cathode rays presumably excited the gas and, on striking glass, caused it to fluoresce, too. It had recently been shown, moreover, that cathode rays (whatever they were!—it would be several more years before they were identified as electrons) could escape the glass tube through a small, thin, aluminum-foil window at the anode end, and then travel a few inches through air. The evidence for this was that certain materials would fluoresce if held near the foil window while the tube was being activated. One such fluorescent substance was barium platinum cyanide.

It is not at all clear what Roentgen was trying to accomplish on the evening of November 8—his will instructed that all of his laboratory notes be burned unread upon his death. It is not even known whether he was using a glass tube with an aluminum-foil window. In any case, the room was darkened, and the tube was completely enclosed with blackened cardboard thick enough to block any light or cathode rays. But Roentgen noticed that a sheet of paper coated with barium platinum cyanide, located a short distance away, would glow while (and only while) the tube was firing—and neither visible light nor cathode rays could be responsible. Most remarkably, when he held a small object between the tube and the screen, the flesh of his hand seemed nearly transparent, revealing the shadows of the bones within.

Roentgen was aware that he might have stumbled onto something entirely new. But might there perhaps be a simple, obvious explanation that he was overlooking? Far more disturbing was the possibility that perhaps he could not trust his own senses. "I . . . believed," he later recalled, "that I was the victim of deception when I observed the phenomenon of the ray."[1] One biographer described Roentgen's anxiety this way:

Could the images on the screen be playing tricks on his mind? Roentgen spent an appreciable amount of time during the next few days verifying that he really was seeing what he thought he was seeing, and that he was not simply suffering from hallucinations. His career as a scientist would be over, his credibility gone. It is easy to understand Roentgen's bewilderment, because he seemed to be observing phenomena that had no known, rational physical explanation. Was this fact or illusion? Roentgen knew his physics literature, and knew that nothing like it had been described before. He worried that he might have become seriously unbalanced. He wrote to his longtime friend, physicist Ludwig Zehnder: "I had spoken to no one about my work. To my wife I merely mentioned that I was working on something about which people would say, when they found out about it, 'Roentgen has surely gone crazy.'"[2]

Over the following weeks, Roentgen stopped all other work and practically moved into his lab. His wife Bertha is known to have expressed serious worry about his behavior, lamenting that her normally devoted husband had become erratic and peculiar. His assistant, whom he locked out of the laboratory, reported that Herr Professor was withdrawn and short-tempered. Roentgen appeared oblivious to their concerns. He repeated the experiment feverishly, varying every parameter that could possibly have a bearing on its outcome. When asked later what he thought upon discovering X rays, he replied, "I did not think; I investigated."[3]

It was not until he produced an X-ray photograph of Bertha's hand (figure 2) that he came to believe that these new rays were indeed real, and that he was not coming unhinged. Regrettably, the photograph had an altogether different effect on Bertha. She had long held a terrifying premonition of an early death, and seeing the resemblance of her hand to that of a skeleton gave her a most unpleasant shock. She never went near her husband's laboratory again.

On December 28, Roentgen submitted a paper describing his findings, "On a New Kind of Ray," to a local scientific journal. Within days, news of the discovery was excitedly picked up by the press and spread throughout the world. The importance of the work was recognized right away, and not just by a few specialists. X rays immediately intrigued scientists in all fields, captured the public's attention on a grand scale, and, beyond all the excitement, provided the medical community with an extremely effective and practical new diagnostic tool. More than a thousand technical and medical papers were published on the subject within the single year following the discovery. For his work, Roentgen was offered a title, which he refused, and received numerous awards, including the first Nobel prize in physics in 1901. He donated the prize money to the University of Würzburg.

Soon after presenting his discovery to the world, Roentgen returned to his former research interests and wrote only seven more papers. In October 1914, he joined ninety-two other professors in issuing a manifesto in support of German militarism, an action that he later regretted. His family lost its wealth and suffered considerable hardship during World War I and the inflation that followed. After a short illness, during which he kept careful records of his own symptoms, Roentgen died in Munich on February 20, 1923.

CHEST X-RAY EXAMINATION OF A YOUNG AIDS PATIENT WITH PNEUMONIA

Alex Roman, a nine-year-old child originally from Vladivostok, was born with hemophilia, an inherited inability of the blood to clot properly. His condition has required regular transfusions of Factor VIII, the missing essential blood component. In the days before donor blood could be adequately screened in Russia for the human immunodeficiency virus (HIV), which is responsible for acquired immunodeficiency syndrome (AIDS), Alex received a contaminated transfusion. The HIV virus invaded his immune system and, by killing off one type of white blood cell (the T-lymphocytes), destroyed much of his ability to combat infections. Alex's physicians in the United States were unaware of this condition until, as he turned six, he began displaying signs of abnormally slow development. His motor skills were poor, and he could not read or count as well as his friends. These and other more obvious symptoms, such as weight loss, lethargy, rashes, and an increase in the number of his fevers, pointed to HIV infection. This suspicion was confirmed with a blood test, which revealed the presence of a specific antibody, directed against the virus, that his body was producing.

Antibodies are proteins (produced by another group of white blood cells, the B-lymphocytes) specifically designed to chemically recognize and then bind to particular "foreign" materials. The combination of an antibody with its antigen then signals other components of the immune system to seek out and attack the intruder. The HIV antibody, in particular, binds to the surface of the HIV virus. Regrettably, the body's immune system is usually not powerful enough to combat effectively a full-scale HIV onslaught.

While detection of the antibody in a blood sample confirms infection with HIV, the seriousness of the infection is gauged by the extent to which the targeted T-lymphocyte population has been depressed by viral destruction. In Alex's case, the T-lymphocyte count had dropped to a critically low level.

Alex began treatment in 1996 with the anti-HIV drugs AZT and DDI, which slow the virus's ability to reproduce itself. His T-cell count rose, and over time his apparent developmental difficulties diminished somewhat. His doctors hoped that he might be one of those fortunate HIV-positive individuals who lead nearly normal lives for long periods of time.

Lately, however, Alex's condition has deteriorated. Last month, he began feeling particularly tired and low-spirited, and three weeks ago he de-

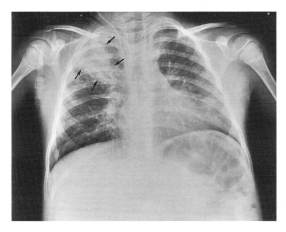
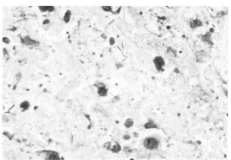

Figure 17 (left). A chest X-ray film of a young AIDS patient at the onset of pneumonia due to tuberculosis. It reveals the lungs, the shadow of the heart, the ribs and spine, and the diaphragm (the sheet of muscle that separates the chest compartment from the abdomen). The lighter, cloudy area indicated by the arrows is strongly suggestive of pneumonia. Figure 18 (right). A sample of sputum showing three tuberculosis bacteria, the thin rods near the center of the photomicrograph. Courtesy of Thomas A. Fleury, Sibley Memorial Hospital, Washington, D.C.

veloped a 102 degree fever. Breathing sounds from the upper right portion of his chest were soft, compared with the rest of the lung, when heard through a stethoscope. This suggested a decrease in airflow in that region. Also, percussion (tapping with the fingers) of the chest produced a duller resonance from that area. It seemed that some abnormal process had filled the upper right region of the lung with fluid.

A radiograph immediately corroborated this suspicion. In the developed film (figure 17), the arrows point to a relatively light and cloudy area, indicating a portion of the lung through which a smaller than normal number of X-ray photons were able to pass—some dense material is there that should not be. The clinical findings and the film together strongly suggested pneumonia, an infection and inflammation of the lung. Normal lung tissue is like a damp sponge, containing mostly air. Here, however, the infected portion of the lung appears to be filled with pus and other fluids. Because of its greater density, lung tissue saturated with these fluids attenuates X rays (removes them from the beam) much more effectively than does healthy lung. The corresponding area on the film therefore appears lighter.

The location of Alex's pneumonia, in the upper lobe of a lung, is typical of pulmonary (lung-related) tuberculosis (TB), the specific form of pneumonia caused by the tuberculosis bacterium. That initial diagnosis can be validated through microscopic examination of a coughed-up sample of sputum (figure 18). While the TB itself can be a very serious matter,

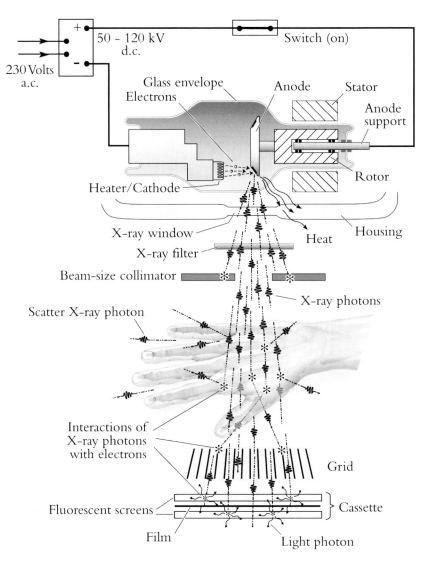

Figure 19. A modern radiographic system. When the exposure switch is briefly closed, as shown here, the high voltage produced by the generator is applied between the two electrodes of the X-ray tube. Electrons that boil off from the negatively charged, white-hot cathode accelerate through the vacuum and smash into the positive anode. There, about 1 percent of their kinetic energy of motion is transformed directly into X-ray radiation. The resulting uniform beam enters the patient's body, and the spatially varying X-ray shadows emerging from it are captured on a sheet of special photographic film within a cassette. The more X-ray energy that makes it through the body and exposes an area of the cassette, the darker the corresponding region of film will be upon development.

its onset indicated, even more significantly here, that the HIV infection had developed into a full-blown case of AIDS.

Alex was admitted to the hospital and given oxygen and physical therapy of the chest. A catheter (a thin plastic tube) was inserted into a vein

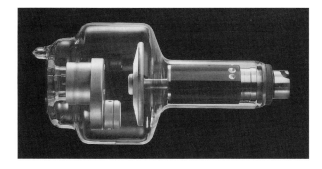

Figure 20. A modern X-ray tube. The cathode assembly, to the left, and the anode and rotor are clearly visible through the glass envelope; the anode is made to spin rapidly by the rotor (supported on bearings) and stator that comprise an induction motor. The tube will be encased within a housing that contains X-ray shielding and also oil for cooling and high-voltage insulation.

to allow intravenous infusion of anti-TB drugs. Drug-resistant TB is an emerging and potentially lethal problem, but fortunately the strain that attacked Alex was not of that sort. After a week of therapy, a new film demonstrated marked improvement. Two weeks later, the chest was completely clear, and Alex's appetite had returned. His physicians have discontinued the AZT, and are beginning treatment with newer drugs (3TC, D4T, and a protease inhibitor) in an attempt to establish control over the HIV.

TAKING AN X-RAY FILM: A SHORT STORY

Despite the development and availability of other important imaging technologies such as computed tomography and magnetic resonance imaging, film radiography remains the most widely employed means of obtaining medical images. It is also, in some regards, the easiest to describe. For both reasons, we shall begin our exploration of clinical imaging with the story of how an X-ray image is formed on film.

And it really is a story, with a proper beginning (the generation of an X-ray beam), plot development (the interaction of the beam with the bones and soft tissues of the patient), and a possibly momentous denouement (the formation of a radiographic image that may—or may not—be capable of resolving a clinically crucial question). The production of an image with a modern radiographic system thus involves three quite separate processes (figure 19):

First, an X-ray tube generates a penetrating, uniform X-ray beam.

Then, various bones and soft tissues of the patient's body absorb and scatter different amounts of the X-ray energy, thereby imprinting an X-ray shadow image onto the previously uniform beam.

Finally, patterns of remnant, unabsorbed X rays emerging from the body expose a radiographic cassette containing a sheet of special photographic film, leading to the formation of a visual image after the film is developed.

The more radiation that reaches any part of the cassette, the darker the corresponding portion of film becomes. In a chest film, for example, a rib lets through relatively little X-ray energy, and thus shows up as a pale band against the dark, opaque surrounding areas of the film that correspond to lung and muscle tissues, which are more transparent to X rays.

Let's examine these three processes in a little greater detail.

Generation of a Penetrating, Uniform X-Ray Beam

The anode is made to spin rapidly during an exposure (causing a faint whir) to spread out the area actually bombarded with electrons—and that helps to keep any region of it from overheating. As you can imagine, getting a white-hot anode within an evacuated vessel to rotate thousands of times per minute, with no normal lubricants available, all the while applying a very high voltage to it, involves some rather fancy engineering footwork.

Our story begins with a nearly uniform beam of penetrating X rays, produced by an X-ray tube and its generator. The generator acts, in effect, like a very high-voltage battery with a timer-controlled on-switch. The evacuated glass or metal X-ray tube contains two metal electrodes, the cathode and anode, which are connected to the negative and positive terminals of the generator, respectively (figure 20). The cathode is a coiled wire filament that is brought to high temperature, so that electrons "boil" off it— but as long as the exposure switch remains off, the electric circuit is open and incomplete, and nothing very interesting happens.

To take an X ray, the exposure switch is activated (closed) for a few hundredths of a second, thereby applying a brief pulse of high voltage (and creating an electric force field) between the two electrodes of the tube. Some of the (negatively charged) electrons that are thermally driven off the (negatively charged) cathode are electrically attracted toward the (positive) anode. They pick up a great deal of speed in their fleeting journey through the electric field—just as a porcelain vase will in the Earth's gravitational force field.

When these high-velocity electrons crash into the anode, roughly 99 percent of their collective energy is dissipated in heating it. The tube is useful for imaging only because as the electrons slam to a halt, the other 1 percent of their collective energy is converted directly into X rays. As noted in appendix A, whenever a charged particle undergoes a rapid change in speed or direction, as happens when an electron crashes into the anode, a portion of its energy of motion is converted into electromagnetic radiation. Energy is not created or destroyed in the process; it simply changes form and radiates away—just as most of the motional energy of the falling vase is expended in shattering it and heating the parts, but a small amount is transformed directly into sound radiation.

An X-ray beam contains photons with a range of energies. These extend up to a maximum individual photon energy numerically equivalent, in standard units known as electron volts (eV), to the voltage setting of the generator. With a generator applying a 90,000-volt drop across an X-ray tube, the most energetic photons will each have 90,000 eV of energy.

Radiant energy produced in this fashion exits through a window in the metal housing and radiation shielding that surround the tube. It then transits an aluminum filter that preferentially removes low-energy photons. (Virtually none of them would pass completely through the patient, so they are diagnostically useless, but they would deposit radiation dose unnecessarily.) The beam is now ready to make pictures.

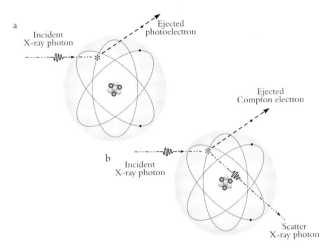

Figure 21. There are two important mechanisms by which diagnostic X-ray photons interact with matter, whether it be tissue within the patient or the fluorescent material of a cassette. (a) In a photoelectric absorption event, the photon imparts all of its energy to an atomic electron. The photon is removed from the beam, the electron is ejected from the atom at high velocity, and the atom is ionized. (b) In a Compton scatter collision, only part of the incoming photon's energy is transferred to an atomic electron; the rest leaves the scene of the interaction in the form of a lower-energy scattered X-ray photon. Either way, X-ray photons are removed from the beam; interactions that take place within the patient's body imprint a shadow image in the X-ray beam. Also, either way, energy is deposited in irradiated materials (patient and cassette); X-ray photons that pass through the patient and strike a fluorescent screen of a cassette produce bursts of light that expose the X-ray film.

What the Patient's Body Does to the X-Ray Beam:
Formation of an X-Ray Shadow

As Roentgen discovered, only a fraction of the X-ray radiation entering any piece of material exits from its far side. Some photons will be either absorbed or scattered by atomic and molecular electrons, instead, and are thereby removed from the beam (figure 21). A hand gives rise to a meaningful X-ray shadow because bone absorbs or scatters more photon energy from a beam than do the surrounding soft tissues.

There are several reasons that one region of the body might be better than another at stopping X rays. As a general rule, the more material there is in the beam path, the more probable it is that any particular X-ray photon will interact with some atom, and thus be culled from the beam. So the thicker the body part that the beam is entering (or the more obese the patient), the less the amount of X-ray energy that makes it all the way through (figure 22).

Likewise, the rate of beam attenuation increases with tissue density. Lung, for example, consists of soft tissue and of spaces filled with air.

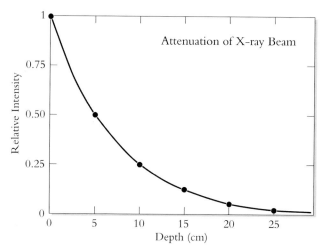

Figure 22. Attenuation of an X-ray beam passing through soft tissue. As ionizing radiation traverses a block of material, roughly the same fraction of what remains is absorbed or scattered in each centimeter. Suppose, for example, that the intensity of an X-ray beam entering the material from the left is 1, and that it falls to $\frac{1}{2}$ in traversing 5 centimeters. At a depth of ten centimeters, only about half of that remains, or $\frac{1}{4}$ of the original beam strength. Likewise, 15, 20, 25, . . . centimeters into tissue, the intensity will be about $\frac{1}{8}$, $\frac{1}{16}$, $\frac{1}{32}$, . . . The beam is said to be undergoing exponential attenuation.

Normal lung is only about one third as dense as muscle or water, so a beam must travel through three times as much of it to lose the same quantity of photons. Conversely, bone is about twice as dense as muscle—a major reason why it attenuates X rays so much more effectively. Because of these differences in density, radiographs normally have little trouble distinguishing muscle or the internal organs from lung or from bone. The contrast among these three is normally very high for a radiograph (figure 23a).

Note that it is the pattern of X rays that have *not* interacted with the body's tissues—have *not* been absorbed or scattered—that exposes the radiographic cassette and thereby affects the film within. So, in a sense, an X-ray image is a negative: the thicker and denser parts of the body produce regions in the developed film that are lighter and more transparent. Conversely, the thinner or less dense the tissues in the beam path, the stronger the emerging beam and the darker the resulting film.

Attenuation of a beam depends also on the chemical makeup of the substances it crosses through. X-ray photons are more inclined (for reasons that would take us too far afield to explain here) to interact with heavier atoms (those with higher atomic numbers). Bone mineral consists largely of calcium and phosphorus atoms, while muscle is composed predominantly of the lighter elements hydrogen, carbon, and oxygen. This

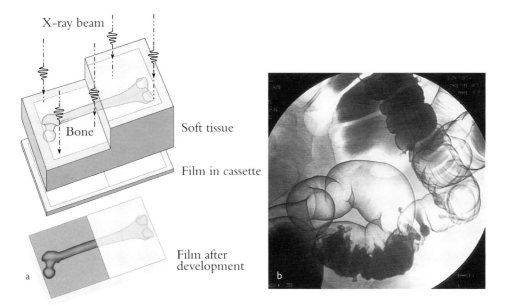

X-ray beam

Bone

Soft tissue

Film in cassette

Film after development

a

b

Figure 23. Contrast is a measure of the extent to which tissues that are anatomically or physiologically different appear so in an image. (a) The contrast of a bone with its surroundings depends on the thickness of the tissue in which it is embedded. (b) A contrast agent can artificially enhance certain features in an image. A swallowed barium "cocktail" helps to outline a portion of the bowel here, for example, and iodine-based contrast agent does the same for blood vessels (see figure 10b). Figure b courtesy of William McCann, South Muskoka Memorial Hospital, Bracebridge, Ontario, Canada.

difference is another source of the high contrast of bone shadows on X-ray films.

The contrast for an organ or particular tissue refers to the extent to which it stands out from the other, nearby tissues in an image (figure 23a). Contrast of a tissue can sometimes be enhanced artificially by altering its physical properties with X-ray contrast agents. Because iodine atoms are very heavy and happen to absorb X rays particularly strongly, blood vessels containing intravenously injected iodine compounds tend to stand out clearly from the surrounding soft tissues. Barium has similar application for the esophagus, stomach, and intestine (figure 23b).

One additional factor that determines how rapidly a beam is attenuated in a material is the effective energy of the X-ray beam itself. The more energetic the photons are on average (somewhat like heavier, hence more energy-laden, bullets), the less likely they generally are to be absorbed or scattered by matter, and the deeper they tend to penetrate into and through it. Thus the *attenuation* rate (the relative amount of intensity lost when a beam passes through, say, one millimeter of material) depends on the beam energy. Not only that, but the way in which the attenuation rate

In the past, contrast agents have been of somewhat limited help in the radiographic search for brain tumors. An ordinary X-ray film of the head usually reveals nothing but bone, even for very bright patients. But in a difficult and often painful procedure, a radiologist could fill the ventricles (the large, interconnecting, fluid-containing cavities that are a normal part of the brain) with a dense liquid

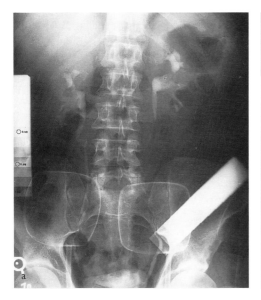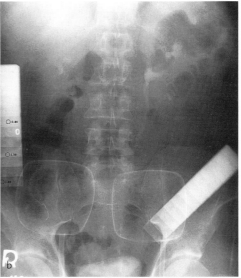

Figure 24. An important, and adjustable, determinant of image quality in radio-graphy is the voltage applied across the X-ray tube by the generator. The image to the left, (a), was made at a lower voltage (70,000 V) than (b), the one on the right (110,000 V). As a result, (a) more clearly shows the two ureters, which are carrying urine (and iodine-based contrast agent) from the kidneys to the bladder. The lower the voltage, the better the contrast, but the greater the amount of radiation dose that is delivered to the patient—one of many trade-offs to be considered in imaging. Courtesy of the American College of Radiology.

contrast agent or a gas, which would make them stand out from the surrounding tissues. Any evident distortions or displacements of them would suggest the presence of something that didn't belong. This was all rather chancy, though—trying to diagnose tumors of the brain without being able to see either the tumor or the brain. Fortunately, the wonderfully revealing pictures produced non-traumatically by CT and MRI have largely eliminated the need for this unpleasant business.

varies with photon energy differs from one material to another. So for a particular study, the beam energy can be selected for the greatest relative differences among the tissues of interest, and thus for best image contrast (figure 24).

Capturing the Pattern of X Rays That Emerges from the Body

In a typical chest radiograph, roughly 99 out of every 100 X-ray photons that enter the body are absorbed or scattered by its atoms, and would thereby (ideally) be removed from the beam. Thus only about 1 percent of the beam's photons pass through the patient unscathed. Embedded in this pale remnant beam, however, is an X-ray shadow image that reflects the spatial distribution of the variously attenuating tissues or other objects within the body.

Along with the faint X-ray shadow emerging from the body, however, are many of the scatter X-ray photons that were created within it. These are heading every which way, and a number of them would strike the cassette and film randomly, adding visual background noise and degrading contrast significantly. Fortunately, much of this scatter radiation can be re-

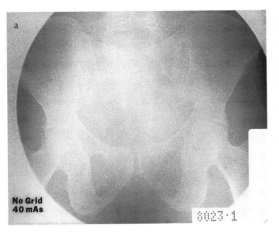 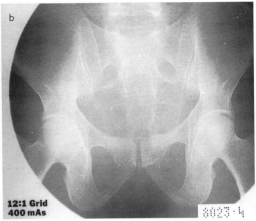

Figure 25. Scattered X rays produced within a patient's body degrade image contrast. (a) Radiograph of a pelvis, taken without a grid. (b) When a grid is used, the contrast is considerably better, but the radiation dose to the patient is higher; to end up with the same average darkening of the film, it is necessary to increase beam output to compensate for what the grid removes. A second trade-off. Courtesy of the American College of Radiology.

moved by an anti-scatter *grid*, which acts like a Venetian blind consisting of thin lead louvers, letting through only those X rays that have *not* undergone scattering within the patient, and are still traveling in their original direction (figure 25; see also figure 19). Selecting as small an X-ray field size as possible also helps, by minimizing the amount of scatter radiation produced in the first place.

Most scatter photons are subsequently absorbed within the body itself, and do not degrade the image.

After passing through a grid, the beam might now be allowed to expose a sheet of radiographic film directly, as is normal practice in dental radiography. Radiographic film is a semi-rigid sheet of plastic coated on both sides with thin layers of emulsion. Emulsion is a dry gelatin within which are suspended vast numbers of microscopic crystals composed of silver and bromine ions plus carefully controlled small amounts of other chemicals (figure 26a). An X-ray photon that strikes a single grain of silver bromide will deposit energy in it and "sensitize" it; during the subsequent chemical development of the film, those individual crystals that were sensitized (but only they) lose all their bromine, and transform into flecks of metallic silver (figure 26b). The remaining, *un*transformed silver bromide crystals are then dissolved and removed from the gelatin during the chemical fixation and washing of the film. In a portion of the film subjected to a higher level of X-irradiation, a greater number of the silver bromide crystals turn into specks of silver metal during development; the processed film will be more opaque to light there, and thus appear darker to the eye.

With routine dental exposures, you clamp between your teeth a tab attached to the small sheet of film. There is no grid or fluorescent screen, but in other regards intra-oral filming is much the same as standard medical radiography.

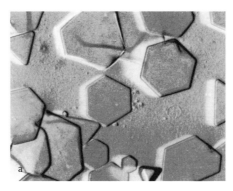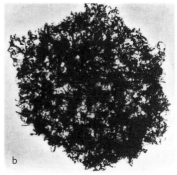

Figure 26. What makes photographic film dark: (a) The active ingredient in film is tiny crystals of (mostly) silver bromide, seen here with the aid of an electron microscope. (b) During the chemical development process, those microcrystals that were sensitized by exposure to X-ray or light photons are transformed into tiny flecks of opaque, pure silver metal, one of which is shown here. The crystals that are not sensitized (and are not subsequently converted to metallic silver) are dissolved and removed from the film during fixation and washing. Courtesy of Arthur Haus, Eastman Kodak Company.

But film is relatively insensitive to high-energy photons, so you have to use a lot of them to create an image, and a fair amount of dose is deposited in the patient. An X-ray image is therefore usually recorded in a more efficient, two-step process. It is first transformed into a pattern of visible light within a radiographic film cassette; it is this visible *light* image that then actually exposes the film within the cassette. A cassette consists of two fluorescent screens, between which is sandwiched the sheet of film (see figure 19). Since a fluorescent screen is so much thicker and denser than a film, many more X-ray photons interact with it. In addition, whenever a single X-ray photon does collide with the fluorescent material, the screen emits a pinpoint burst of *thousands* of visible-light photons, which can transform a cluster of many (not just one) silver bromide crystals into grains of pure silver. For these two reasons, much less X-ray exposure is required to darken the film by the required amount when fluorescent screens are being used, and the radiation dose to the patient may be tens or even hundreds of times lower.

The price to be paid for this reduction in patient dose is some loss of resolution. In a cassette, the light has room to diffuse a little within a translucent intensifying screen before reaching and striking film, producing a tiny cluster of silver grains. This noise introduced by the finite size of the clusters (a phenomenon known as quantum mottle) will diminish the sharpness achievable—as with Seurat's dabs of paint. The thicker the screen, the more efficient the screen is at capturing X-ray photons, and the lower the patient dose—but the more a burst of fluorescent light can spread out before forming clusters of silver grains, the larger the resulting dabs will be and the poorer the resolution. A range of screens and film speeds allows selection of the optimal sharpness-dose balance for any particular study. If exquisite detail is not needed, you can choose a "faster" screen that leads to less patient dose. And that is generally held to be a good thing.

WHAT THE X-RAY BEAM DOES TO THE PATIENT'S BODY: RADIATION DOSE AND RISK

As was shown in figure 21, an X-ray photon that scatters from or is absorbed by an atom normally ejects an electron from it, thereby ionizing it. Within the patient's body, in particular, an X-ray photon will knock an electron out of almost any atom or molecule it interacts with. Unfortunately, that's not the end of the story. As it travels at high speed through tissue, a newly liberated electron will itself collide with hundreds or thousands of atoms that happen to lie along its path, ionizing them as well. Even a single high-energy photon absorbed or scattered in tissue can thus end up ionizing hundreds or thousands of biomolecules. All of these newly ionized molecules will briefly have too few, or too many, electrons on them, and that may render them highly unstable and chemically reactive. This reactivity can become problematic if some of the molecules affected in the process are the DNA of your genes.

The activities of every one of the fifty or so trillion cells in your body are largely under the control of the cell's own copy of your particular, unique set of DNA molecules. A strand of DNA is much like a long chemical ticker tape, carrying complex genetic directions that the cell requires to perform its appointed biochemical tasks. The DNA turns chemical reactions on and off, in effect, in response to chemical messages coming in from the rest of the cell, and this feedback mechanism orchestrates and regulates all cellular activities.

When an X-ray photon collides with an atom in a cell, there is a *slight* chance that a DNA molecule will be ionized, thereby becoming unstable and reactive. The DNA may then begin a complex sequence of chemical changes that could result, eventually, in significant alteration of its information content, rather like randomly punching a few extra holes here and there in a ticker tape (figure 27). Fortunately, such an error will almost never be of any consequence. The effect on the cell's operations may be negligible, or the cell may be able to catch and repair the error, or it may simply die. Indeed, it is through the intentional killing of tumor cells in this fashion, without wiping out too many nearby healthy cells in the process, that radiation therapy can combat certain kinds of cancers.

Occasionally, though, the radiation-induced genetic misinformation

Patient motion is another important contributor to the *un*-sharpness of an X-ray film. So, too, is the finite size of the focal spot in the X-ray tube. The focal spot is the minuscule region on the anode from which the X rays actually originate—and just as the shadows cast by a floodlight are fuzzier than those from a tiny bulb, the millimeter or so dimensions of a real focal spot will cause a slight blurring that a perfect point source of X rays would not.

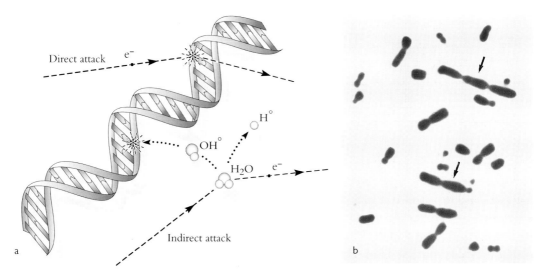

Figure 27. Radiation damage to a DNA molecule. (a) The DNA can be directly ionized by a passing high-velocity electron, or attacked indirectly by a chemically reactive molecule known as a free radical, such as the OH° and H° radicals produced when a water molecule (H_2O) is broken apart. (b) DNA is packaged as chromosomes, which part of the time are visible under the microscope. For a female, each should appear like a tiny letter X. This particular set of chromosomes, from a hamster cell irradiated with X rays, contains two that are misformed, direct evidence of radiation damage. Figure b courtesy of James B. Mitchell, National Institutes of Health.

will direct an otherwise stable cell to make a copy of its DNA and then to divide into two nearly identical daughter cells. The same erroneous DNA command to replicate and divide will be passed on to both daughters, moreover, and then to *their* progeny, and to all future generations of cells. This condition of uncontrolled cell proliferation may result in a malignant tumor or, if the affected cell is a precursor cell for white blood cells, in leukemia. Alternatively, if there is radiation damage in an egg cell in a woman's ovary, or in sperm in a man's testicle, faulty genetic information may subsequently manifest as an abnormality in their offspring. Finally, if the damaged DNA belongs to a cell in a fetus, it may induce a developmental deformity or other form of harm in the child. In any of these three cases, the results can be catastrophic.

I must emphasize that the probability of such serious cellular changes actually occurring as a result of a normal radiographic examination is *extremely* small. A patient's radiation risk from an appropriately prescribed diagnostic film would almost inevitably be much, much lower than the far more certain risks from forgoing the examination and suffering the medical consequences. Virtually all experts would agree that if a radiological study is clinically called for, its benefits will greatly outweigh the risks, and that the odds strongly favor the patient who undergoes it. Nonetheless, the prudent physician and medical staff minimize the exposure of the patient, and of themselves as well, to *nonproductive* radiation. Indeed, a number of state and federal public health policies and regulations exist to encourage this.

To help put the risks in perspective, we should remember that we live in a sea of ionizing radiation already. Each day we are bombarded by cosmic rays from outer space. Likewise, virtually all things on Earth (including us!) contain at least trace amounts of naturally occurring radioactive materials, and we are continually exposed to their ionizing radiation. As it happens, the incremental radiation dose from a chest X ray, for example, is equivalent (with respect to the estimated hazard) to what we receive from natural sources in a matter of days. It is also much less than the increases in natural background radiation you would experience in flying across the country a few times, or in moving for a year from, say, Jersey City to Aspen, in the Colorado Rockies, where the protective blanket of the atmosphere is thinner. Still, where would you rather be?

ASSESSING RADIATION RISKS

Risk, in its normal usage, refers to the possibility that something bad may happen, and it takes into account both the probability of occurrence and the extent of potential harm. A mildly dangerous event may appear too risky if the odds of it happening are not small; and even an extremely improbable event may seem like a poor risk if it could lead to terrible results.

Psychologists have found that the level of anxiety or outrage that people feel about a hazard depends strongly on its source. Humanmade hazards tend to be less acceptable, and may actually seem much more perilous, than equivalent dangers that occur naturally. Likewise, people perceive as more risky those threatening situations that are imposed without consultation or consent, rather than experienced voluntarily. And the level of perceived risk increases if the hazards seem unfair or have no visible benefits. It is ironic, and at times leads to tragic consequences, that the perceptions of risks that commonly determine people's beliefs and actions are often totally at odds with the real risks that confront them.

Fortunately, it is sometimes possible to compare hazards quantitatively. Such is often the case in medicine, where it is standard practice to seek quantitative measures of the risks and benefits associated with various diagnostic and therapeutic procedures. In radiology, of particular

---

concern is the possibility that the ionizing radiation used in a radiological procedure might itself inadvertently give rise to a cancer. Assessing the likelihood that this might happen requires two quite separate kinds of information. One is the amount (dose) of radiation actually deposited in the irradiated tissues during the procedure. The other is the risk (probability of cancer induction) per unit of radiation delivered. The product of these two factors provides an overall estimate of the risk:

$$Risk = (Dose) \times (Risk/Dose)$$

First, we must quantify the radiation dose. There are several standard measures of ionizing radiation, but we shall stick with units widely used in risk assessment in the United States: the rem and the millirem (1 mrem = 0.001 rem). How much radiation does a rem represent? Background radiation provides a reasonable yardstick: a person typically receives the equivalent of a uniform, whole-body dose of about 300 mrem (0.3 rem) each year from unavoidable natural sources such as cosmic rays and radioactivity in soils and rocks.

The greatest source of manmade radiation is medical procedures. But while some of the exposures involved in radiation therapy may be quite large (thousands of rems, sometimes over a significant part of the body), those from diagnostic procedures are not. The dose from a standard chest radiograph, for example, ranges from about 20 millirem in the skin at the point where the beam enters the body, to a few percent of that amount where it exits and exposes the radiological cassette. In other words, the average dose within the chest from a properly taken radiograph is comparable to what the same volume of tissue gets from natural background radiation over a matter of days—and, of course, the volume of tissue exposed is much less.

So much for the *Dose* part of our equation, and now on to the *Risk/Dose* term. It has been known for years that large amounts of ionizing radiation can cause cancer (and very high doses can kill a person outright). But at the low dose-levels normally encountered in most X-ray examinations (tens or hundreds of millirems, and only to part of the body), the number of cancers caused by radiation is so very small that we have no way to assess the risks directly. The best available evidence on cancer induction, in fact, comes from epidemiological studies of people who have received considerably higher doses, such as the survivors of the atomic blasts at Hiroshima and Nagasaki. Studies of ninety thousand of the surviving inhabitants of those cities, begun shortly after

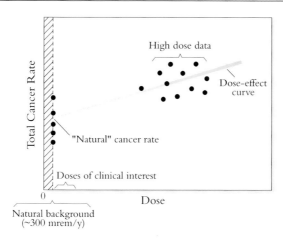

Figure 28. The only firm data on radiation-induced cancers among humans have been culled from studies of people exposed to relatively high doses. Most public health officials assume, in devising public health policy, that the risk declines linearly as exposures diminish down to the lower-dose levels encountered in medical imaging. It is also assumed that the straight dose-effect line continues all the way down to zero dose—which is to say, even a small dose has some small risk associated with it. The evidence in support of this linear, no-threshold hypothesis is controversial, and the field is one of active research and debate. One important complicating factor is the 300 mrem of background radiation we are all exposed to every year from natural sources; normal variations in background can be greater than diagnostic doses, making the statistics of the induction of cancers by radiation extremely difficult to pin down.

the end of the war and still ongoing half a century later, indicate that people who received doses significantly higher than background level were more likely to be stricken with cancer eventually.

At the higher doses of these studies, it appears clear that the probability of cancer induction is proportional to the dose received (figure 28). But there are severe difficulties in trying to extend the argument from these doses, for which a fair amount of data exists, down into the low-dose region relevant to diagnostic imaging. Quite simply, we do not know for sure how hazardous small additional amounts of ionizing radiation really are. Possibly we never will, because the data are so hard to obtain. A major difficulty is that the few cancers that the small amounts of diagnostic radiation may be inducing are indistinguishable from the vast numbers that arise spontaneously—or that are being caused by the sea of natural background radiation around us. There are probably so few of them, moreover, that they cannot be discerned by statistical analysis with any assurance. This is not to imply that medical people think the potential hazards are in any way unimportant; we just cannot detect them, assuming that they are present.

Still, many researchers feel that the available epidemiological information and the results of laboratory studies of irradiated animals and cell cultures strongly suggest that at relatively low doses, cancer risk is at least roughly proportional to the radiation dose, and that there is no dose threshold below which exposures are totally safe. It is commonly assumed, moreover, that the value of *Risk / Dose* is the same at low doses, give or take a factor of two or three, as at higher doses, where it *can* be estimated from the epidemiological data. The validity, or error, of this "linear, no-threshold" assumption is the subject of much scientific debate (along with a fair amount that is not so scientific). Indeed, it is fully recognized that very small amounts of radiation exposure—that is, below some threshold level—may be harmless. Still, the linear, no-threshold assumption is widely adopted by public health physicians and officials as a prudent, conservative working hypothesis upon which to build public health policy and regulations for protecting patients, medical staff, and members of the public from radiation dangers. (This view has been endorsed by the National Academy of Sciences, the International Commission on Radiological Protection, the National Council on Radiation Protection and Measurements, and other major scientific advisory bodies.)

The generally accepted estimates of *Risk / Dose* for lethal cancers are in the vicinity of 5×10^{-4} (5 / 10,000, or 0.0005) per rem. That is, the statistics suggest that if 10,000 people all received a uniform, whole-body dose of one rem (1,000 mrem), then about five of them would die prematurely because of a cancer induced by the radiation (with the disease typically appearing ten or more years after the exposure). With a lower dose, or if only a part of the body is exposed, it is assumed that the risk would be correspondingly lower.

SPECIAL CONSIDERATIONS FOR MAMMOGRAPHY

Breast cancer strikes one of every nine women in the United States, and more than 180,000 new cases of the disease are diagnosed each year. Fortunately, if malignant tumors are caught early, when they are still small and localized, the five-year survival probability may be better than 90 percent. The problem is that the smaller a tumor is, the harder it is to detect.

While some small masses can be picked up with regular clinical breast exams by a physician or through breast self-examination, mammography may reveal their presence even before they can be felt. Indeed, in 1997 the National Cancer Institute and the American Cancer Society agreed that

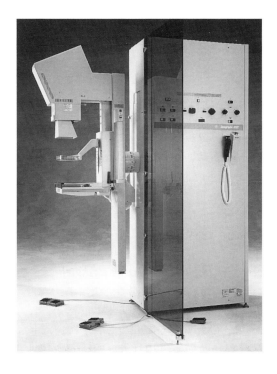

Figure 29. A dedicated mammographic system, with specialized mammographic X-ray tube and generator, breast compression device, antiscatter grid, cassette, and film. Courtesy of General Electric Medical Systems.

"mammography screening of women in their 40s [and older] is beneficial and supportable with the current scientific evidence."[4] The challenge has been to improve the effectiveness of screening mammography for women under age fifty, whose breast tissues tend to be denser and harder to image. The situation may change with the improved sensitivity and selectivity that will come with the further development of digital mammographic systems, and possibly of other imaging technologies (in particular, MRI and ultrasound). Of course, close surveillance is generally appropriate for women of all ages who have a family history of the disease or other risk factors.

Mammography must be able to reveal not only subtle differences in the density and composition of breast tissue, possibly indicative of the existence of an abnormal mass, but also the presence of calcifications, tiny flecks of bonelike material that may be of diagnostic importance. Thus high contrast, good spatial resolution, and low noise are all required. The response of the imaging system, moreover, must be flexible enough to accommodate not only the low-intensity beam emerging from the tissue near the chest wall, but also the much greater number of X-ray photons that pass through the side and front edges of the breast. And last, but by no means least, the dose should be kept low to minimize both radiation risk and patient anxiety.

Each of these objectives may be easy to achieve separately, but meeting all of them simultaneously is no simple task. A modern dedicated mammographic unit is therefore designed to achieve the best possible balance among these somewhat conflicting requirements (figure 29). Typically, such a system is made up of a specially designed mammographic X-ray tube and generator, a breast compression device, a grid, and a cassette with only one fluoroscopic screen and film with emulsion on only one side of the plastic sheet. Contrast among the radiologically similar soft tissues of breast is enhanced by imaging with very low-energy X-ray photons; attenuation is higher and beam penetration is poorer, which is not desirable, but relative *differences* in attenuation between different tissues, such as tumor and normal breast, are accentuated, which is crucial. Compression of the breast between a pair of parallel, flat, X ray–translucent paddles spreads out the tissues to a uniform thickness for better visualization; this generally increases image contrast, prevents blurring from patient motion, and even reduces tissue dose.

CASE STUDY

A MAMMOGRAM THAT REVEALS A SECOND MALIGNANT BREAST TUMOR

Mrs. Elizabeth Israel, a fifty-five-year-old businesswoman and mother of two teenage children, has an annual physical, performs monthly breast self-examinations, and had one set of mammograms taken at age fifty. None of this revealed any abnormality, but her medical history is of concern. She menstruated from ages twelve to fifty; her first child was born when she was forty; and her older sister (but no other members of her immediate family) has had breast cancer. The lengthy menstrual experience, her advanced age at the birth of her first child, and, most important, the history of breast cancer in a close family member all suggest that she is at greater than average risk for the disease.

Mrs. Israel recently noticed that the nipple of her left breast seemed to be pulled inward. In examining her, her gynecologist felt, behind the nipple, a hard mass the size of a small marble that could be moved about easily. The other breast appeared normal. No skin of either breast was inflamed, nor were there any other palpable lumps in her breasts, or in or below her armpits. Of the three most likely causes of this kind of lump in the breast—a benign growth, a cyst, or a malignancy—the inverted nipple suggested the presence of cancer.

Such a suspicious change in a breast calls for a biopsy, in which a small sample of the tissue of concern is excised and examined in the pathology laboratory, but mammograms of both of Mrs. Israel's breasts were taken first. These, it was hoped, would provide additional pre-biopsy information suggesting whether the mass was indeed cancerous. The films would also make possible a search for other irregularities not detected by phys-

RADIATION RISK FROM A MAMMOGRAM

We can use the numbers discussed earlier to provide a *rough* estimate of the radiation risk from screening mammography. The dose to the skin of either breast at the point of beam entrance might be 500 to 700 millirem per film, with an average dose throughout the radiation-sensitive, milk-producing glandular tissue of 0.1 to 0.15 rem. Two views are taken of each breast.

Let us assume that for a whole-body X-ray exposure, *Risk / Dose* is 5×10^{-4} per rem. From our risk equation, the estimated *Risk* is

(2 films) x (0.15 rem per film) x (5×10^{-4} risk per rem) x (0.05),

where the 0.05 is an additional, empirically obtained, approximate multiplier that accounts for the fact that only the breasts are being irradiated, not the whole body. This estimated risk of 7.5×10^{-6}, about one in a hundred thousand, is comparable to the likelihood of dying in a crash when driving your car around town for a short while or flying across country—which is to say, *extremely* small. It should be noted that the use of other reasonable numbers in the product could give a result that differs from this by as much as an order of magnitude (a factor of ten). If a woman has a dozen or so mammograms over the course of a lifetime, the estimated cumulative risk is on the order of 1 in 10,000. For an older woman, this is much smaller than the probability that she will be stricken with a breast cancer that could have been detected at an early stage with a mammogram.

The odds favor those women who have appropriate routine mammograms.

ical examination. Finally, they could assist the surgeon who would actually perform the biopsy.

In the mammography suite, Mrs. Israel expressed some reservations about the compression of her breasts. The radiographer acknowledged that there can be discomfort for some women, but showed her two films (kept on hand for this purpose) of another patient's breast. These had been taken with gentle, and subsequently with firmer, compression; the differences in clarity and contrast were convincing, even to an untrained eye (figure 30). Compression is especially important for large breasts like Mrs. Israel's, where the image contrast tends to be inherently lower.

With the left breast held firmly between the two compression paddles of the mammographic X-ray machine, a film was shot from each of three

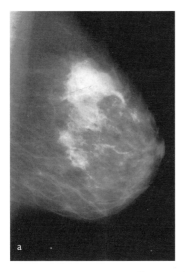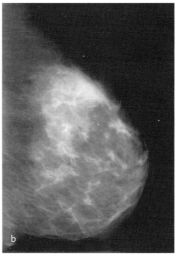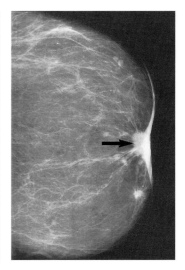

Figure 30 (left and center). The effect of compression on mammograms: (a) With gentle compression, there appeared a region on film suggestive of a tumor. (b) When the compression was tightened, the apparent tumor vanished, and no biopsy had to be performed. Courtesy of William McCann, South Muskoka Memorial Hospital, Bracebridge, Ontario, Canada.   Figure 31 (right). A mammogram, in which the nipple is inverted, pointing into the breast. Behind the nipple is a clearly evident tumor, indicated by the upper arrow. A second area of concern appears below the tumor.

different angles (one is shown in figure 31). Behind the inverted nipple, a typical spiculated (i.e., with outreaching, invasive tendrils) tumor with tiny calcifications can be seen. These features are all suggestive of malignancy. A second area of concern appears just below the palpable lump. The three mammograms taken of the right breast were normal.

Several days after the first mass was discovered, a surgeon removed the two lumps found on the mammogram. A pathologist examined sections of the two masses under a microscope and determined that both were indeed malignant (figure 32). The specimens also showed that the surgeon had excised a good margin of healthy breast tissue around each tumor; it was therefore unlikely that bulk cancer had been left behind in either area of the breast. The normal appearance of a sample of lymph nodes taken from under the left armpit, moreover, suggested that the disease had *not* spread to the lymphatic system, so no further surgery was performed. This type of limited operation, in which most of the breast is left intact, is known as a lumpectomy.

After the surgical wound had healed sufficiently, Mrs. Israel began a course of radiotherapy, in which a high dose of ionizing radiation (many thousands of times greater than that used in making a mammographic film) is deposited in the breast. This is intended to kill any remnant tumor

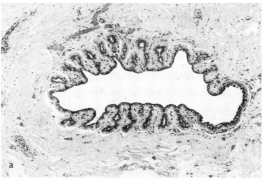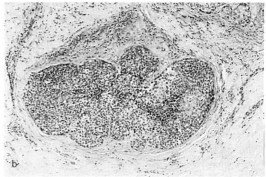

Figure 32. Photomicrographs of a milk duct in (a) normal, and (b) cancerous breast tissue. Courtesy of Thomas A. Fleury, Sibley Memorial Hospital, Washington, D.C.

that might have escaped excision during surgery, and also to eradicate any other cancers that had not shown up on the mammograms. Studies of large numbers of cancer patients with her type and extent of disease indicate that such women who undergo lumpectomy and then radiation treatment have the same rates of survival as those who have the entire breast removed (mastectomy). That being the case, Mrs. Israel had decided that the cosmetic advantages of lumpectomy plus radiation outweighed her concerns about risks from leaving the breast in place.

Further laboratory tests revealed that the tumors were non-aggressive and estrogen-receptor positive; that is, the growth of this type of tumor is stimulated by the normally occurring female hormone estrogen. So after completion of the radiotherapy treatments, she began receiving the drug tamoxifen, which blocks estrogen's stimulation of tumor growth. This treatment will continue for up to five years. It was felt, however, that the benefits of a full course of chemotherapy would be marginal in her case.

Mrs. Israel's prognosis is excellent. There is a good chance that the disease will not recur and that she will live out a normal life. And she has promised herself that from now on, she will have mammograms taken regularly.

Chemotherapy involves injecting specific toxic materials into the bloodstream, to kill any remaining cancer cells (which may be more vulnerable to certain kinds of chemical damage than are most normal cells), including those that have broken free of the primary tumor and lodged elsewhere in the body. The toxins may also destroy sensitive but important healthy cells, however, and treatment can lead to unpleasant side effects. Recent advances in chemotherapy have made some of the process much easier to endure.

3

Shadows on Television, Live
FLUOROSCOPY

When Roentgen placed his hand in an X-ray beam and beheld the bones of his fingers on a fluorescent screen, he was creating the first fluoroscopic image. Within months, medical practitioners around the world were employing essentially the same approach in their clinics.

In the early days, they did this in a darkened room by projecting a beam through the patient, with the X-ray image appearing directly on the screen. But they first had to adapt their eyes to the dark for perhaps half an hour and, even then, the images were faint and of low contrast. So with the steady flow of improvements to conventional film radiography, medical fluoroscopy fell largely by the wayside. By midcentury, perhaps its most widespread remaining application was in the thousands of shoe-fitting fluoroscope units scattered around the country (figure 33). Apparently these contraptions were sources of great amusement ("Lemme look, too!"), but they subjected customers (primarily children) and sales clerks to considerable radiation and sometimes serious damage, and were actually quite useless in the search for comfortable footwear.

THE RENAISSANCE OF FLUOROSCOPY

Because of two major advances in electronics—television and the X-ray image intensifier—fluoroscopy has enjoyed a renaissance and is once again a standard means of producing medical images.

Ever since Samuel Morse telegraphed "What hath God wrought!" from

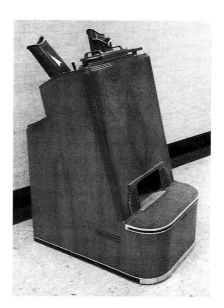

Figure 33. Several people could simultaneously view the bones of the feet by means of this ancient shoe-fitting fluoroscope. Courtesy of Oak Ridge Institute for Science and Education.

Washington to Baltimore on May 24, 1844 and, three decades later, Alexander Graham Bell's assistant heard the first intelligible words sent by telephone, "Mr. Watson, come here. I want you," people dreamed of transmitting pictures, too, over wires or through the air. It was not until 1923, however, that a patent for a television camera (the iconoscope) was filed. Television broadcasting began in London in 1936, and in the United States five years later. Spurred on by the wartime effort to perfect radar, by the 1950s television had acquired sufficient spatial and contrast resolution, low noise, and reliability to allow millions to share the joys of Howdy Doody and the Mickey Mouse Club, and even to display visual medical information.

Nearly as memorable as Bell's summons was the reaction, soon thereafter, of Pedro II, Emperor of Brazil, to a demonstration of the new wonder: "My God! It speaks Portuguese!"

The other critical technical advance was the development, specifically for radiology, of the X-ray image intensifier—a vacuum tube device that can transform a life-sized pattern of X rays emerging from a patient into a small, bright visible-light image. The optical image it generates can be captured by a still or motion picture camera, and for some purposes this alone offers big advantages over standard film radiography (see figure 9). But only when the image intensifier was combined with television did fluoroscopy begin to reach its full potential.

By feeding the output image from an image intensifier tube into a video (television) camera, one can display clearly, on a nearby or remote TV monitor, radiological procedures as they are happening. The sharply visible patterns of an injected radiographic contrast agent flowing through blood vessels can be observed while they occur, for example—not after long minutes of waiting for motion picture film to be developed. The movement of swallowed contrast agent past a constriction in the throat can be watched as it takes place and viewed again and again from videotape. Real-time viewing has also proved invaluable in setting bones and in surgically removing shrapnel and other foreign bodies. It is also practically indispensable in planning the radiation therapy treatments of cancer patients.

Wedding the image intensifier to television provided a powerful new way to view the interior of the body in real time, and it brought fluoroscopy wholly back into the diagnostic fold. In so doing, it made possible novel approaches to treating patients, as well. Now the physician can make repairs to the body while viewing it, like a surgeon, but with a minimum of surgical trauma. In a procedure known as balloon angioplasty, for example, she can position the tip of a special catheter at the site of a partial blockage in a blood vessel, and then inflate a balloon in the tip, forcing open the constriction—all possible because she can manipulate and operate the balloon while observing it live, with real-time fluoroscopy.

Long after fluoroscopy had reestablished a central position for itself in the imaging clinic, a third technology, that of the computer, elbowed its way into the fluoro suite. The signal from a video camera can be converted to digital electronic form, which provides for entry into the realm of digital image processing, storage, and communication. Perhaps the most striking result of combining fluoroscopy with computers has been digital subtraction angiography (see figure 10). In the study of blood vessels, DSA eliminates the obscuring and confusing X-ray patterns produced by all other tissues, a great benefit that we will explore in the next chapter. But we'll stay with nondigital fluoroscopy, for now, and begin to examine its workings with a case study.

CARDIAC CATHETERIZATION FOLLOWING A HEART ATTACK

CASE STUDY

Eliot T. Stearns is a hard-driving fifty-five-year-old, the owner of a financial periodical. He has been on medications for fifteen years to control his blood pressure and cholesterol level, but admitted he was frequently too busy to take them. Despite repeated warnings from his physician, he smoked two packs of cigarettes a day, was sixty pounds overweight, and had little, but intermittently vigorous, exercise. His father died of a heart attack in his early forties.

Over the course of six months, Mr. Stearns began to notice an unusual heaviness and pressure in his chest after walking up a flight of stairs. The sense of constriction became progressively more noticeable, even at night as he lay in bed. One evening he awoke with an agonizing crushing sensation in his chest and sharp pains in his left arm and jaw, caused by an inadequate supply of oxygen to the heart muscle. He felt nauseated and was sweating profusely. In the emergency room, the admitting physician immediately recognized the classic signs of angina and a probable heart attack. An electrocardiogram (EKG), which monitors the electrical signals generated by the heart as it functions, confirmed this diagnosis, showing irregularities that pointed to damage to heart muscle. In addition, blood tests revealed elevated levels of certain enzymes indicative of injury to cardiac muscle.

The heart is a pump that pushes freshly oxygenated blood coming from the lungs through the arteries to the tissues of the body, and drives the returning, oxygen-poor blood back through the veins to the lungs. As one ages beyond the middle years, irregularly shaped plates of yellowish fatty material (plaque) can build up on the inside walls of arteries. This can lead to their hardening (atherosclerosis), and may also act as seeding points for the formation of blood clots (thrombosis); plaque buildup can severely obstruct blood flow. In Mr. Stearns's case, a blockage had occurred in one or more of the coronary arteries that carry oxygen-rich blood from the lungs and heart directly to the cardiac muscle itself. As a result, a portion of the heart muscle, starved of oxygen, was dying.

The blood also transports carbon dioxide from the tissues back to the lungs, where it is released to the atmosphere. Tissue cells slowly "burn" sugars and other carbon-based molecules in oxygen, producing chemical energy and heat, and CO_2 as a waste by-product. Plants, by contrast, harness energy from sunlight to cycle the CO_2 in air back into oxygen and energy-rich carbon molecules.

The patient was given an oxygen mask to increase the concentration of oxygen in the blood reaching the heart muscle tissue still marginally alive; drugs to dissolve the clot in the coronary artery; nitroglycerine to dilate that artery (and the others) to facilitate blood flow through it; and morphine to alleviate the pain. After five days of stabilization in the coronary intensive care unit, during which he experienced recurrent chest pain, Mr. Stearns underwent a cardiac catheterization to determine how much plaque had accumulated and the extent to which the coronary arteries had been blocked.

In the cardiac catheterization laboratory, which is equipped for both surgical and radiological procedures, a catheter was inserted into an artery in his groin. Under fluoroscopic navigation, it was directed up into the aorta (the principal artery carrying freshly oxygenated blood from the lungs and heart to the rest of the body) to a point just short of the heart itself. There, the tip of the catheter was mechanically guided into one of the coronary arteries. An iodine-based contrast agent was injected rapidly through the catheter, causing the artery to stand out briefly against the background of soft tissues (figure 34). A partial blockage of the flow of blood was clearly evident on the video monitor.

Mr. Stearns's cardiologist and radiologist, finding what they had anticipated, attempted to reduce the amount of blockage by means of balloon angioplasty. The catheter was pushed a little further into the coronary artery, to the site of the blockage, and a balloon at its tip was filled with a

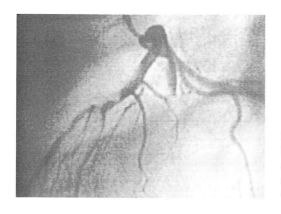

Figure 34. With radiographic contrast agent highlighting the vessel, a blockage in a coronary artery is clearly evident in this cardiac catheterization study. Courtesy of Kevin Nealon, Chevy Chase, Md.

mixture of water and contrast agent. The expanding balloon pushed outward against the plaque built up inside the arterial wall, in the hope that this would widen the channel. Repeated inflations of the balloon failed to improve blood flow significantly in this coronary artery, unfortunately, or in any of the others.

The next step to consider, in terms of its greater risk and cost, was bypass surgery, in which the plugged coronary arteries would be surgically removed and replaced with healthy blood vessels taken from elsewhere in the body. But because of the patient's recent heart attack and poor general condition, his doctors felt that surgery at this time would be too stressful to his heart. Mr. Stearns was therefore treated with nitroglycerine patches to dilate the blood vessels and alleviate the angina, and with beta-blockers to slow the heart rate. He also took aspirin to reduce the tendency of his blood to form clots, which might break loose and lodge elsewhere—perhaps causing another heart attack or, if a blockage occurred in the brain, a stroke.

Six months later, Mr. Stearns remained unable to work because any exertion still led to angina. Sixty-five pounds lighter and free of cigarettes, he underwent coronary bypass surgery. In an eight-hour operation, his body was cooled (to decrease its need for oxygen), and his heart was stopped (to facilitate the extremely fine work of sewing delicate blood vessels together), its pumping action temporarily taken over by a mechanical pump. The diseased arteries were replaced with clean veins taken from his legs.

Mr. Stearns returned to the office three months later. He now takes aspirin and medications for cholesterol and blood pressure regularly, and doesn't go near cigarettes. Through a low-fat diet and a carefully arranged exercise program, including thirty laps daily in a pool, he has kept the weight off. Having transferred his most demanding problems to younger and hungrier members of the firm, he is in psychotherapy and taking an antidepressant to help him deal with the adjustments in his life. Lately he has been noticeably more relaxed, and he tells his family and friends that he feels better and happier than he has in years.

FLUOROSCOPY = X-RAY TUBE + IMAGE INTENSIFIER + TELEVISION

In fluoroscopy, the X-ray tube is left on or pulsed rapidly, so that the physician can view a live, continuously changing image, rather than a radiographic snapshot, frozen in time. With some systems, the X-ray tube points upward from beneath the patient table, and the image intensifier tube views downward from above. Alternatively, the X-ray tube and image intensifier can be at opposite ends of a rigid "C-arm" support, as in figure 35, that can be rotated about one or more axes. Either way, the image intensifier tube faces directly into the X-ray beam, with the patient in between.

The Image Intensifier

An image intensifier (figure 36a) is a marvelous device that can transform a body-sized pattern of X rays into a small optical image, introducing little distortion or noise in the process. When detail is important, the tube's output screen can be photographed directly with a still camera or, primarily for cardiac studies, with a cine (movie) camera. But for the immediacy and flexibility of real-time viewing, the image is fed into a video camera.

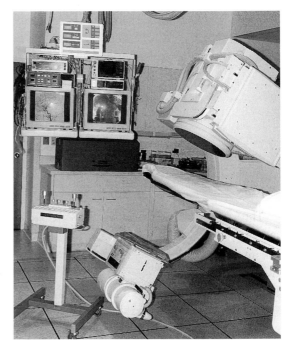

Figure 35. Fluoroscopy is like radiography, except that the X-ray beam is repeatedly pulsed or left on continuously, and the image receptor is an image intensifier, rather than a film cassette. Here, the X-ray tube (below the table and to the left) and image intensifier (upper right) are at the two ends of a C-arm support that can be rotated about one or more axes. The output screen of the image intensifier tube is normally viewed by a video camera.

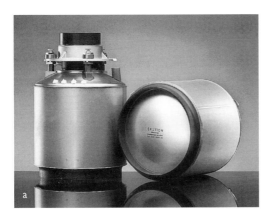

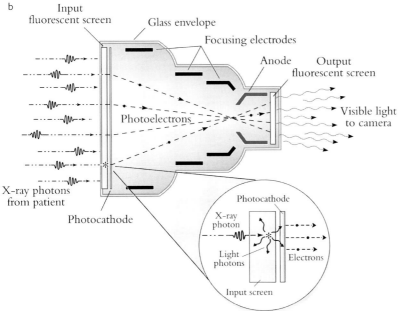

Figure 36. (a) An image intensifier is an electronic vacuum tube that transforms the life-sized X-ray shadow pattern emerging from a patient into a small, very bright optical image. This, in turn, can be picked up by a still camera, a movie camera, or, for real-time viewing, a video camera. (b) The principal components of an image intensifier are the input fluorescent screen plus photocathode combination, the anode, the focusing electrodes, and the output fluorescent screen. Figure a courtesy of Philips Medical Systems.

The four principal components of an image intensifier tube are shown in figure 36b: the large (15–35 centimeters across) input fluorescent screen, the interior surface of which is covered with a thin veneer of photosensitive metal (the photocathode), from which electrons can easily be dislodged by visible light; the electron-focusing electrodes; the anode; and the small (3 cm in diameter) output fluorescent screen.

During an exposure, an X-ray photon that managed to pass through the patient strikes the image intensifier tube's input screen, producing a tiny burst of light (X ray–stimulated fluorescence). Light photons from the screen eject electrons from the adjacent photocathode (photoelectric effect), and these newly liberated photoelectrons are drawn immediately toward the anode. That is, a life-size X-ray shadow produces a life-size visible-light image, which, in turn, gives rise to a life-size pattern of photoelectrons that begin moving toward the anode. The X-ray image information is now carried in, and represented by, the spatial configuration of these electrons. As they accelerate toward the anode, the electrons are squeezed closer together by the focusing electrodes, which shrinks the image they convey by a factor of five to ten. On striking the small fluorescent output screen at high velocity, each electron produces a bright point-flash of light (electron-stimulated fluorescence). The net result is an optical image at the output screen with human anatomy appearing much as it does in an ordinary developed X-ray film, only much smaller. But the image intensifier tube's output image is thousands of times brighter than the one originally produced on its input fluorescent screen, and of a size suitable for recording by a film or television camera.

The Television Link

A TV system usually consists of a video camera for acquiring the image; a monitor for display; an information transmission channel connecting the camera to the monitor; and possibly a videotape recorder for storage (figure 37a). With the closed-circuit television found in most imaging departments, the transmission channel consists of electrical cables; the monitor may be in the same suite as the imaging device, but it could also be elsewhere in the hospital, or even more distant. For wireless transmission, signals are sent from a microwave or radio frequency transmitter, perhaps by way of earth-orbital satellite, to a receiver. Either way, an optical image (such as from an image intensifier tube) is captured by the camera, transformed into an electromagnetic signal, transmitted and received as such, and finally converted back into a visual display at the viewing monitor.

A vacuum tube video camera is designed to convert a two-dimensional optical image into an electrical voltage that varies with time, called the *video signal*. The visual image from an image intensifier, say, is projected by glass lenses onto the front surface of the thin, photosensitive "target" inside the camera tube, as in figure 37b. Meanwhile, a narrow beam of electrons rapidly and repeatedly traces out a raster pattern (closely spaced parallel lines) on the *back* side of the target. The electrical properties of the target material are sensitive to light, such that wherever on the back of the target the scanning electron beam happens to be striking, the voltage coming from the target at that instant is proportional to the amount of light focused at the corresponding point on the (illuminated) opposite side. As the electron beam scans a pattern of light that varies in two spatial dimensions, in effect, the image is encoded in the form of a video signal voltage that varies accordingly over time.

A vacuum tube display reverses the process, transforming the received video signal back into an optical image (figure 37c). An electron beam within the tube scans its fluorescent display screen, following the same raster pattern adopted by the video camera. At the same time, the video signal coming from the camera is being detected by the receiver and applied to the display tube's grid; this electrode acts like an electron spigot, regulating the number of electrons striking the fluorescent screen at that instant—hence the level of brightness there. The video signal voltage, which varies with time, is thus translated back into a two-dimensional spatial pattern of parallel lines of varying brightness, somewhat like an engraving, as you see in figure 37d.

The resolution of a system with a television link is limited mainly by the electron beam scan pattern. Some medical fluoro systems employ the raster pattern of American broadcast television, in which a single frame (image) is made up of 525 parallel lines of spatially modulated brightness. Modern fluoro TV systems, and good computer monitors, commonly use about 1,000 lines per image (as will commercial high definition television, HDTV), and some even achieve 2,000 lines per frame. In general, though, the resolution lies in the 1 to 0.3 mm range (i.e., objects any closer together than that are not seen as being separate), depending on the equipment, and that is about ten times poorer than for film radiography. Fortunately, the resolution of fluoroscopy is perfectly adequate for many tasks.

Recently developed solid-state optical devices such as the charge-coupled device (CCD) camera used in camcorders, and the flat-panel liquid crystal displays (LCD) found in virtually all laptop computers, work quite differently from the conventional vacuum tube cameras and monitors described above, but they can produce pictures suitable for many clinical applications. Because they tend to be much smaller and lighter, require no high voltages, waste less energy as heat, do not emit electromagnetic radiation that could interfere with electronic medical equipment, and are more rugged, they (or other solid-state devices) are likely to displace their vacuum tube aunts and uncles in the clinic over time.

Solid-state X-ray image receptors are also being developed that can directly transform a pattern of X rays into a voltage signal. Making use of the specially advantageous electrical and mechanical properties of thin films of amorphous (glasslike, noncrystalline) silicon or selenium, such devices would replace the combination of image intensifier tube plus video cam-

Putting it slightly differently: suppose the camera's scanning electron beam encounters a spot on the target where the other side of the target is brightly illuminated; the camera instantaneously sends out a message to the grid of the monitor, instructing that the electron beam in the display tube deposit a bright spot at the corresponding point on its fluorescent screen. The two electron beams are made to sweep out the same raster pattern and in synchrony.

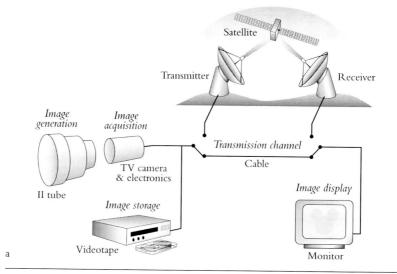

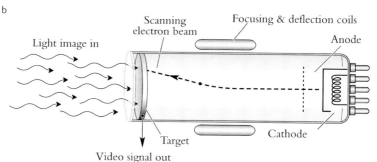

Figure 37. Television. (a) A rudimentary TV system consists of video camera, communications channel, and display monitor, with videotape for signal storage. (b) An optical image entering a vacuum tube video camera produces a pattern of illumination on the front of the camera's photosensitive "target." An electron beam sweeps out a raster pattern on the back side of the target. The camera generates a video signal voltage that, at any instant, is proportional to the brightness of light at the point on the front of the target across from the point on its back where the electron beam happens then to be striking.

era. In so doing, they would be able to provide better resolution, less visual noise, and all the benefits of digital technology, which will be discussed in the next chapter.

EVER VIGILANT:
THE NEED FOR QUALITY ASSURANCE

X-ray tubes and generators, image intensifiers, video cameras, monitors, and all the other bits and pieces that might go into a medical imaging unit are usually stable and reliable. As with any other complex machine, though, a tune-up or part replacement is occasionally needed. So an es-

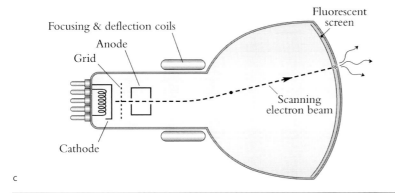

c

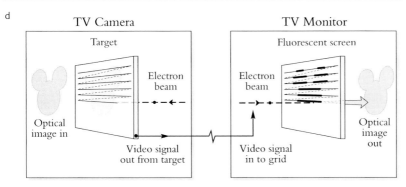

d

Figure 37, continued. (c) In a vacuum tube display monitor, the electron beam aimed at the fluoroscopic front screen of the tube sweeps out the same raster pattern that the camera uses. The incoming, time-varying video signal is amplified and applied to the grid, which controls the number of electrons striking the fluorescent screen per second, hence the brightness of the scanning point of light. (d) Summary of the TV process: A camera encodes a two-dimensional pattern of light as a video signal voltage that varies over time; a monitor transforms the time-varying video signal voltage back into a two-dimensional pattern of light.

sential aspect of the operation of any medical imaging facility is a rigorously implemented quality assurance (QA) program, designed to ensure that the images produced are diagnostically as useful as possible and that the risks to the patients and staff are minimal. A QA program may be required by state and/or federal regulations, but whether voluntary or mandated by law, adhering to it is wise and cost-effective, and works in everybody's best interest.

QA programs are usually established and managed by specially trained Ph.D.- or M.S.-level physicists who have chosen to apply their skills in the medical setting. Some elements of the program are carried out daily or

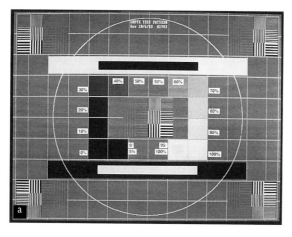
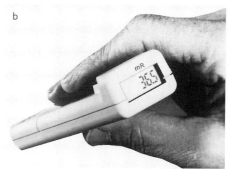

Figure 38. A quality assurance (QA) program involves a number of measurements and tests for image quality and radiation safety. (a) This test pattern was introduced into a television system electronically (not through viewing with a video camera) to check aspects of monitor electronics. (b) Virtually everyone directly involved in producing X-ray or gamma-ray images wears a film badge, which keeps track of the amount of radiation received over the course of a month or so; excessive darkening indicates higher than normal exposure(s). Shown here is a pocket dosimeter, which immediately records doses deposited over minutes or hours, and which is carried by a worker who might be exposed to significant amounts of radiation. Courtesy of Nuclear Associates.

Medical physicists are also largely responsible for the selection and installation of new equipment, technical aspects of the development and oversight of clinical procedures, and some of the teaching of radiologists-in-training.

weekly by the radiographers who normally operate the imaging equipment in patient examinations, but the more complex checks are performed by the medical physicists. Scheduled QA tests can catch many partial equipment failures before they become serious difficulties. As an X-ray tube ages, for example, its anode becomes a bit cratered at points where it was briefly overheated, causing its focal spot to enlarge and reducing radiograph resolution and sharpness. Likewise, some links within the television chain can slowly deteriorate and subtly degrade the signal, leading to slightly lower image contrast, or perhaps adding a pinch more visual noise. Such changes can add up and slowly diminish the system's ability to reveal clinically important image patterns, unless staff can discern and correct the problems early (figure 38a).

The radiation safety component of a QA program ensures that the amount of radiation produced by an X-ray machine is sufficient to provide clinically useful images, but that the dose to the patient does not exceed that amount. Similarly, it is important that the exposures borne by the staff, who work around patients and the equipment day after day for years on end, be monitored and kept to a minimum (figure 38b). Some exposure is inevitable, but following a few commonsense rules (stay as far as possible from the source of radiation, while still being close enough to carry out the job properly; minimize exposure time; use proper radiation shielding; always wear a film badge radiation sensor) and adhering to the other elements of a standard radiation safety program minimize risks to patients and staff.

A BARIUM SWALLOW
FOR ESOPHAGEAL CANCER

Ibn Zuhr (Abenzoar) of Seville, who died in his seventh decade in A.D. 1162, was among the most influential clinicians of medieval Islam. His *Practical Manual of Treatments and Diet* was translated into Latin and Hebrew and highly regarded even in the Christian West. Ibn Zuhr describes one patient's condition as "beginning with mild pain and difficulty in swallowing, and going on gradually to its complete prevention."[1] This is perhaps the earliest reference to the diagnosis and treatment of a tumor blocking the esophagus, the tube that carries food and liquids from the throat to the stomach. Ibn Zuhr dealt with such cases by mechanically forcing open the constriction in the patient's throat and by administering nutritive enemas. Although things are done differently now, the disease is still difficult to control.

Real-time fluoroscopic viewing was put to good use in two quite different ways in the diagnosis and treatment of Paula Neruda, a fifty-three-year-old sportswriter. She has smoked two packs of cigarettes a day since high school and has consumed the better part of a pint of gin most evenings since her husband and son were killed by a drunk driver a decade ago.

Half a year ago, she began having trouble swallowing, and she occasionally experienced the sensation of food sticking in her throat. Over the past two months she has lost twenty pounds, mainly because of difficulty in eating. At the insistence of her daughter, she turned to her physician for medical attention.

In a thorough physical examination, Mrs. Neruda's mouth, throat, head, and neck appeared normal. But a sample of stool revealed blood, commonly indicative of a tumor in the gastrointestinal tract. Her recent history and this new finding were consistent with a diagnosis of cancer of the esophagus, a disease associated with heavy smoking and drinking.

It may happen, with cancer, that pieces of the primary tumor break off and are carried by the bloodstream to distant parts of the body, a process called metastasis. Metastases to the liver or the lymph nodes (common sites for the dissemination of the disease) may cause them to enlarge and seem lumpy. Mrs. Neruda's abdomen was soft, the liver felt normal, and no swellings were detected in the lymph nodes of the neck—all indications

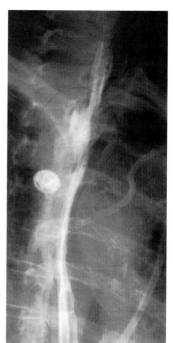

Figure 39. A barium swallow. As the patient swallows the barium contrast material, fluoroscopy reveals a constriction in the lower part of the esophagus. Also visible is an area where a part of its wall has degenerated so much that contrast material can move partially through it. The radiation oncologist has circled the area of known and suspected tumor. This view is from the back, and at an oblique angle. Courtesy of James A. Deye, Inova Fairfax Hospital, Fairfax, Va.

that if cancer were indeed the problem, it may not have spread much yet.

A barium swallow was performed to confirm the presence of a tumor and to pinpoint its location. While she was observed under fluoroscopic television and intermittently filmed by the radiologist, Mrs. Neruda drank a glass of barium-containing X-ray contrast material, a thick, chalky liquid. A major constriction in the esophagus was readily apparent (figure 39), as was an area where the disease had eaten through the esophageal wall, allowing contrast material to spread out. The patient displayed a marked inability to move any swallowed substances past the constriction. The fact that the image outline was immobile during her attempts to swallow suggested that the cancer had invaded the muscles of the esophagus and was interfering with their normal function.

It is usually not possible to make a definitive diagnosis with images alone. A tissue sample, needed to confirm the presence of cancer, was therefore obtained soon after the barium swallow. With the patient sedated, an endoscope was passed down her throat, as in figure 16, and a brush at its end was rubbed against the suspected tumor area. Later that day in the pathology lab, the sample was examined under a microscope and seen to be cancerous.

Esophageal cancer is an extremely serious disease, commonly fatal. Localized radiotherapy treatments can sometimes contribute to a cure, and can often at least improve quality of life for a while. The cancerous tis-

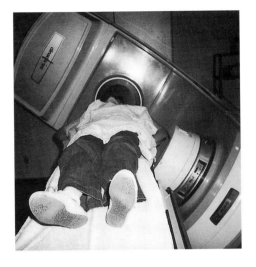

Figure 40. A radiotherapy treatment linear accelerator, or linac, produces a beam quite different from that of a diagnostic machine—the energy of the X-ray photons may be a hundred times greater, and the intensity thousands of times higher. Here, the beam is aimed at the patient's esophagus, and enters from the left posterior. Courtesy of Jack Abarbanel, Alle-Kiski Oncology Center, New Kensington, Pa.

sue is bombarded with the high-energy X-ray radiation produced by a medical linear accelerator (linac), as seen in figure 40. This linac beam, which is significantly more penetrating and delivers thousands of times more radiation than the levels used in diagnostic imaging, will kill cancer cells and may shrink the tumor considerably. In the hope of reducing her problems with swallowing, Mrs. Neruda accepted the advice of her physicians that she undergo radiation therapy, possibly followed by surgery.

FLUOROSCOPY IN RADIOTHERAPY

The objective of radiation therapy is to subject the tumor to heavy irradiation and thereby destroy it, but at the same time not cause an unacceptable level of damage to any essential organs nearby. It would be of little help to eradicate a tumor of the esophagus if the spinal cord were severed in the process. So it is imperative not only that the tumor receive a lethal dose, but also that as little healthy, critical tissue as possible be exposed to high levels of radiation. Radiation treatments are therefore preceded by extensive planning.

Preliminary clinical considerations, including the results of a CT study, indicated that the appropriate treatment for Mrs. Neruda's cancer should be a standard one. First, a pair of large-area therapy beams would irradiate, from the front and back for specific periods of time, the diseased tissues and the surrounding areas of possible spread. In a second phase of treatment, three smaller beams would converge on the tumor region only, to provide a radiation "boost."

Treatment planning for the boost consists largely of selecting the

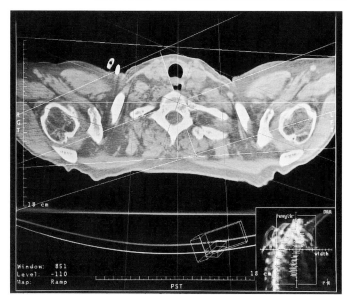

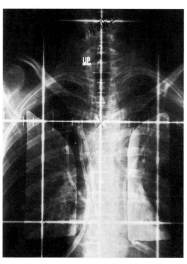

Figure 41 (above). Radiation therapy treatment planning. The physical arrangement of the linac radiation beams for a three-field boost treatment for an esophageal tumor. (The anterior beam exposes the supine patient from above, and the left and right posterior obliques enter through the shoulder blades.) The air passageway, the esophagus, and the spinal cord within the vertebral body are easily seen. To the lower right is a small fluoroscopy-like image constructed out of CT information, a beam's-eye view for one of the posterior oblique fields. The numerous short horizontal lines indicate where the radiation oncologist outlined both the spinal cord (which must be carefully protected) and the region of the esophagus at risk (which must be given a high dose). Courtesy of James A. Deye, Inova Fairfax Hospital, Fairfax, Va.   Figure 42 (above right). Beam's-eye view. One of the three final radiographic films taken during simulation of the boost treatment of the esophagus. The three display what will be the fields of view of the three selected treatment beams, and help to ensure that no critically sensitive organs are being overexposed. Courtesy of James A. Deye, Inova Fairfax Hospital, Fairfax, Va.

three best angles (based largely on computer-generated maps of predicted radiation dose deposition within the body) and calculating the three beam-on treatment times (figure 41). It begins with the "simulation": the patient lies on the table of a specialized fluoroscopic device, the simulator, whose motions can exactly mimic those of the linac that will be used for the actual treatments. Simulation thereby provides a fluoroscopic view of the tumor and surrounding tissues as they would be seen by the linac's X-ray beam. Guided by CT and simulator studies and by the computer-generated dose maps, the radiation oncologist and treatment planning staff settle on what they consider to be the three best treatment beam orientations and sizes—ideally, covering the tumor, but little else, in the high-dose, beam crossfire region. Then the simulator (now acting like an ordinary X-ray machine) shoots three corresponding radiographic films (figure 42). These can be compared later with films taken during the treatment itself, with a brief pulse from the linac providing the imaging X-rays, to ensure that the treatment beams have been aimed correctly.

Following simulation and the other aspects of her treatment planning, Mrs. Neruda came to the radiotherapy department every weekday for four weeks. After the radiotherapy technicians positioned her precisely on the table of the linac, the machine bombarded the target area for a minute or so, from each of the two or three chosen angles, with large amounts of high-energy X rays. During the course of the treatment, recently developed chemotherapy drugs were administered to sensitize the tumor to the radiation.

Mrs. Neruda's treatments seemed to be highly successful. The irradiation managed to kill many of the cancer cells within the tumor region while causing only minimal damage to the surrounding healthy tissues. The radiation-plus-drugs combination shrank the tumor's volume by more than 90 percent, which significantly reduced the amount of surgery needed later to finish the job. With the tumor apparently fully gone after surgery, and with no detected metastases, the treatment may well have effected a complete cure.

But the use of sensitizing drugs with radiotherapy is new, and it is too early to judge their effectiveness; microscopic traces of the disease may possibly remain hidden elsewhere within her body. So Mrs. Neruda and her loved ones will have to endure the wrenching uncertainties of this terrible disease for the foreseeable future.

4

Shadows in Computers
GOING DIGITAL

The speed and computational power of personal computers have been sky-rocketing over the past few decades, and the cost per arithmetic operation has been plummeting. The widespread availability of sophisticated, low-cost PCs and minicomputers has been inspiring extraordinary developments in clinical medical imaging—and what we are seeing now may be only the beginning.

A BRIEF HISTORY OF COMPUTERS

We are the early participants, some have suggested, in the third great transformation of civilized life. The Information Revolution is upon us, and it may well have as profound an impact on human affairs as did the advent of steam-driven industry in the mid 1700s, and the creation of permanent communities and agriculture 12,000 years ago. But the seeds of the Information Age were planted long before those of the earliest domestic grains—they simply required the right conditions to germinate.

People have been computing ever since they discovered fingers. Piles of pebbles and sticks helped the first humans keep track of important matters like the numbers of animals in herds, or days until the next full moon. Scratches on hide, wood, or stone served the same purpose with greater permanence and portability, and eventually led to the invention of written numbers—presumably long before pictographs were devised in Mesopotamia and Egypt, around 3000 B.C., to represent spoken language.

The abacus, perhaps the simplest instrument usable for serious calculations, came into being in Asia more than 5,000 years ago. (Not until the Middle Ages did it find its way to the Arab world and Europe.) A skilled operator can rapidly add, subtract, multiply, and divide sizable numbers, and the device is still widely used in commerce in some parts of the world.

Blaise Pascal nudged open the era of automated computing with his invention of the mechanical calculator in 1642. Pascal's father, an employee of the French tax service, passed his days endlessly grinding out and checking arithmetic calculations by hand. Young Blaise, an extraordinarily gifted mathematician then in his twentieth year, came to his father's relief by envisaging and building a calculating machine that could produce such computations speedily, accurately, and tirelessly. A man of far-ranging interests, Blaise subsequently demonstrated that pressure is transmitted equally in all directions by a fluid (Pascal's Law), played a central role in formulating the mathematical theory of probability, and then retired, at the age of thirty-one, to an ascetic life of contemplation and religious writing.

A device that displayed the flexibility of a true computer, the Analytical Engine, was designed in 1833 by the English mathematician Charles Babbage. Steam-powered and employing binary arithmetic, the Engine could be programmed to solve arithmetic problems. Input and output were to be performed with punched-hole cards, which had recently been invented to allow mass-production looms to weave complex patterns into cloth. Unfortunately, the technology of the time could not achieve the fine tolerances required for the Engine's many metal parts; Babbage's machine was not finished, and his work was forgotten until his papers were rediscovered shortly before World War II.

About the time Babbage's ideas resurfaced, Howard Aiken at Harvard and engineers at IBM began collaborating in the construction of an electromechanical device something like (but in some ways less sophisticated than) the Analytical Engine. The Mark I, driven by the war effort and completed in 1944, weighed five tons, was interwoven with 500 miles of wire, and used more than 3,000 mechanical relay switches. Controlled by a sequence of punched-hole instructions coded on paper tape, the Mark I could carry out three additions or subtractions per second, only a little faster than a person with a desk calculator. This computing machine didn't exactly operate at warp speed, but once under way, it required no human intervention, did not grow weary, and made no mistakes—unless some misguided bug ventured between the contacts of a relay at an inopportune time.

The first totally electronic, general-purpose calculating device was the Electronic Numerical Integrator and Calculator (ENIAC). Designed and constructed by J. Presper Eckert and John Mauchly at the University of Pennsylvania, the ENIAC was used extensively toward the end of the war to produce artillery firing tables. Covering 1,500 square feet and containing 18,000 vacuum tubes, it could compute a thousand times faster than its electromechanical counterparts, executing 5,000 arithmetic operations per second. It, too, suffered frequent bugs, but of a different sort—vacuum tube failures.

The EDVAC, successor to the ENIAC, included the final essential feature of a fully modern computer: a memory that stored not only data, but also the instruction set (program) needed to handle that data. Now instructions themselves could be manipulated just as readily as input data. The happy outcome of this was the possibility of self-modifying programs, wherein the result of a current calculation can affect subsequent calculations and decisions.

From then on, the evolution of computer hardware has been largely a matter of improving (albeit almost beyond recognition) on this design. Machines from the late 1950s were built with transistors (invented in 1947 at AT&T's Bell Labs), much smaller, cheaper, cooler, and more reliable than vacuum tubes. Systems of the 1960s employed integrated circuits, single chips of silicon on which were constructed increasing numbers of interconnected transistors and other electronic components. Computers were still very big, very complex, and confined to large, dedicated centers run by highly trained and experienced personnel.

But then, just as the massive mills and looms of eighteenth-century factories had spawned the small motors that now drive CD players, washing machines, and air conditioners in houses everywhere, likewise the monster mainframes manned by technology's high priests began moving over to make way for PCs operated by you and me. In 1971, the Intel Corporation introduced the 4004, an integrated circuit they marketed as a "microprogrammable computer on a chip." The 4004 contained 2,300 transistors, ran at about 100 kilohertz (several thousand times slower than today's PCs!), had as much capability as the ENIAC, even though it was no larger than a postage stamp, and was affordable. Intel's 80286 microprocessor, released a decade later, was about the same size, but contained sixty times as many transistors. The Pentium chips of the 1990s contain millions—and the computers built around them are now indispensable in countless offices and homes throughout the world.

Lately, parallel processing, in which a number of coupled microprocessors are directed at the same task simultaneously, has been providing means for the realistic modeling of weather behavior, long-term climate change, and other highly complex processes, carrying out computations that were barely imaginable only a few years back. Fast random access memory (RAM) has been growing at a similar pace; whereas chips storing a few tens of kilobytes were considered hot stuff a decade ago, today people think in tens of megabytes. Assuming that the trend of the past two decades continues, gigabyte RAM will be available in a few years. But as they say, you can never be too bright, too wise, or have too much memory.

We've also witnessed spectacular advances in software and interconnectivity. In the early years, only people who were thoroughly versed in the intricacies of their own particular machines could prepare programs for them. To make its commercial computers more user-accessible and to make programs transportable from one device to another, in 1957 IBM released the first higher-level language FORmula TRANslating program; although FORTRAN is still employed in the scientific community, other programming languages have found widespread general acceptance, such as C++ and Java. Application programs written in these languages, but with the nontechnical user in mind, now leave operators of word and image processors, spreadsheets, databases, and games virtually unaware of the underlying layers of software that keep everything functioning in a smooth and coherent fashion (most of the time).

Recently, computers have been learning how to talk to one another. In the past, most of their nonscientific uses have been oriented toward manipulating documents by means of application programs—you call up a word or image processor to create and modify text or pictures. Likewise, a spreadsheet or database management system allows you to manipulate vast amounts of numerical data, lists of names, and so on. Now, however, people are focusing on the extraordinary flexibility and reach of computers in acquiring and communicating information. This focus originated within the Department of Defense at the end of the 1960s, when its Advanced Research Projects Agency (ARPA; now the Defense Advanced Research Projects Agency, DARPA) set about interconnecting a large university community by way of telephone lines. From the ARPAnet grew the Internet, the World Wide Web, and search engines and browsers to help us find our way through it all. Today, people anywhere with laptops and the necessary know-how have access to virtually all knowledge from all public sources, and great power to disseminate their own ideas to others.

Where all of this will lead in the long run is anyone's guess, but I am reminded of what Ken Olsen, the founder and president of Digital Electronic Corporation, said in 1977: "There is no reason for any individuals to have a computer in their home."[1] Maybe he was ruminating on the widely circulated opinion of Thomas Watson, chairman of IBM, of some years earlier: "I think there is a world market for maybe five computers."

With that, it's time for a case study.

DIGITAL SUBTRACTION ANGIOGRAPHY OF A BLOCKED ARTERY

In fluoroscopy, the X-ray energy that passes through a patient falls on the input screen of an image intensifier tube. The image intensifier transforms the life-size pattern of X-ray shadows into a bright, small, corresponding optical image that, in turn, is usually viewed by a video camera. The resulting video signal can be made visible on a nearby or distant TV monitor, and stored on videotape. But the power and flexibility of fluoro can be extended greatly if the continuously varying (analog) signal voltage from the camera is digitized (converted into a digital signal) and fed into a computer.

One important clinical application of the resulting digital fluoroscopy is in the imaging of arteries and veins by means of digital subtraction angiography (DSA). With DSA, the computer obtains and stores fluoroscopic images of an anatomic region immediately before and after a radiographic contrast agent (which strongly absorbs X rays) is injected into the patient's bloodstream. It then subtracts one image from the other, point by point, and the resulting "difference image" shows practically nothing except the blood vessels that contain contrast agent.

Bill Garrison, a vibrant ninety-seven-year-old Bostonian and a fiery, lifelong crusader against social injustice, still has excellent vision, but recently he experienced temporarily blindness in his left eye. His sight returned during the day, and he assumed that the problem was only an ordinary manifestation of the aging process, but he visited his ophthalmologist anyway.

On examination, the eyes themselves appeared normal. The pulsing in the left carotid (the primary artery on that side of the neck), however, was considerably weaker to the touch than in the right carotid. The stethoscope applied to the left carotid revealed a bruit (whooshing sound), moreover, characteristic of the turbulence of blood that is flowing through a narrow stricture. A likely explanation of all the symptoms was an intermittent blockage of the slender artery serving the retina of the left eye. The obstruction was probably caused by emboli (pieces of plaque or clotted blood) occasionally breaking off from an unhealthy portion of the inner wall of the carotid, upstream. This diagnosis could be supported through Doppler ultrasound (described in chapter 7), or magnetic resonance angiography (MRA, chapter 8), or digital subtraction angiography of that artery. The clinic's only MRI machine was in the process of being replaced, and the technologist and the radiologist who normally handled the ultrasound were both home with the flu, so that left DSA. DSA is more invasive and expensive than the Doppler or MRA, but it does the job.

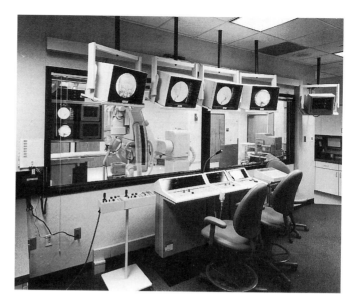

Figure 43. A digital subtraction angiography suite as seen from the control room. With DSA, the output voltage signal from the video camera of a fluoroscopy unit is digitized and fed into a computer. Courtesy of Nuclear Associates.

Under mild sedation, Mr. Garrison was wheeled to the special procedures suite of the radiology department (figure 43). The radiologist performing the examination threaded a guide wire and catheter through the skin and into the femoral artery of his leg, up the leg, and into the aorta, all under standard fluoroscopic guidance. Finally, he skillfully maneuvered the tip of the catheter into the carotid.

The study began by generating and digitizing a fluoroscopic image of the region of interest, and storing it in computer memory (see figure 10). Iodine-based X-ray contrast agent was then injected, and an "after" image immediately obtained. This revealed the vessels that contained the contrast agent, intermixed with a complex of patterns caused by bones and other soft tissues. The subtle details of importance are totally lost in all the confusion.

The "before" and "after" images differ only where contrast material is present. Subtracting them from one another generated the "difference" image, which is virtually blank except for blood vessels that now contain contrast agent (figure 44). This subtraction process eliminates almost all of the shadows made by the background tissues, leaving behind a remarkably clear, high-contrast view of blood vessels alone.

With DSA, a constriction was easily located, but fortunately it was not excessive; the carotid artery was only about 40 percent occluded with plaque. Apparently Mr. Garrison's symptoms would occur whenever a small blood clot—formed on the rough surfaces of the plaque that caused the narrowing in the carotid artery—broke off and flowed into the tiny retinal artery, temporarily plugging it. He was therefore treated with as-

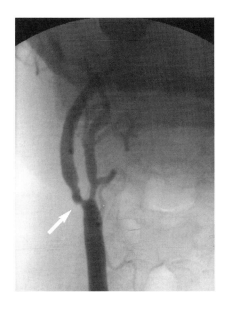

Figure 44. A DSA study of the principal arteries of one side of the neck. The arrow indicates the bifurcation of the common carotid into the inner and outer carotids. Narrowings (stenoses) are visible in both of them, just above fork. See also figure 10. Courtesy of Mohsen Gharib, Suburban Hospital, Bethesda, Md.

pirin and another drug to reduce the likelihood of clot formation. Because of the patient's age, his doctors decided not to submit him to the trauma of surgery unless the situation worsened significantly.

DIGITAL IMAGING VERSUS PAINTING BY NUMBERS

How does an image get into a computer in the first place? The name of the game is digitization, and in its simplest form, digitizing an image is just the converse of painting by numbers.

BITS AND BYTES

A computer thinks and communicates in bits. A bit (for binary digit) is the smallest quantity of information that a computer can process, store, or transmit. It is exactly what is needed to respond to a single yes-no question. "Is it raining?" can have only two answers ("sort of" doesn't count), and the correct one can be supplied with one bit of data. "Is it raining, and is it cold?" requires a two-bit reply. Number of bits is totally unrelated to significance. It might take a million bits to store a trash novel, while a single zero or one in the wrong place conceivably could start a war—or at least crash your PC at the wrong time.

A computer's microprocessor and memory consist of millions of interconnected, microscopic electrical switches built into a silicon chip. These are binary switches, with two possible states of being: shut or

---

open, on or off. These states can be represented by the two English words *yes* and *no*, or by the pair of numbers 1 and 0. A single zero or a one then conveys one bit of information.

Combinations of bits can be used not only to answer multiple yes-no questions, but also to represent numbers, letters of the alphabet, and abstract symbols and concepts. This requires the use of codes, or conventions, to translate ideas and symbols into strings of bits and back again—and the basis for the codes used in computers is the binary number system. A computer is designed to operate with programs and input data expressed in binary numbers.

A connected sequence, or block, of precisely eight bits is called a byte. In nearly all applications, a computer will manipulate bytes rather than individual bits. A simple word-processing program, for example, might assign one byte to each upper- and lower-case keyboard character, with a good number of bytes left over for other symbols.

Suppose we want to modify that famous old World War I black and white photograph of Bill Garrison in his Sopwith Camel, and show him landing next to a 747. We install all the necessary art and design software into a PC, and attach some sort of electronic image acquisition device, such as a scanner or a CCD camera, and point it at the photo. The system starts off by partitioning the image into an imaginary mosaic of many very small picture elements, or *pixels*, each with a unique numerical *pixel address* that indicates its spatial location, as in figure 45. The optical input device and computer would chop the image into an array of adjacent squares, in effect, and then number them sequentially in a raster pattern—like numbering the positions of the characters and spaces as you read from this page. Our photo-imaging unit then views and measures the degree of darkness in each pixel, and translates it into a numerical *pixel value*. The entire image can thus be represented and stored in memory as a long listing of pairs of numbers: the pixel addresses and corresponding pixel values. Now we're ready to use a graphics program to play with the image—in this case, excising the biplane and inserting it into a digitized shot of JFK Airport.

Digitizing a radiographic film is done essentially the same way. Let's say a surgeon in San Diego needs to study a patient's film taken and archived last month in New York City—and she needs it right away. Once the required radiograph is located (which could take considerable time, since it's buried in a stack of films in Dr. Jones's office, and he's off on a month-long lecture and golf tour of Burkina Faso), it is entered into a digitizer, as

Keeping track of the brightness or color while scanning an image along a raster path is a simple and effective way to transform a two-dimensional spatial image into a (one-dimensional) time-varying voltage or a sequence of numbers. Recall from chapter 3 that a vacuum tube video camera does much the same thing by sweeping its electron beam in a raster pattern, as does a video monitor tube.

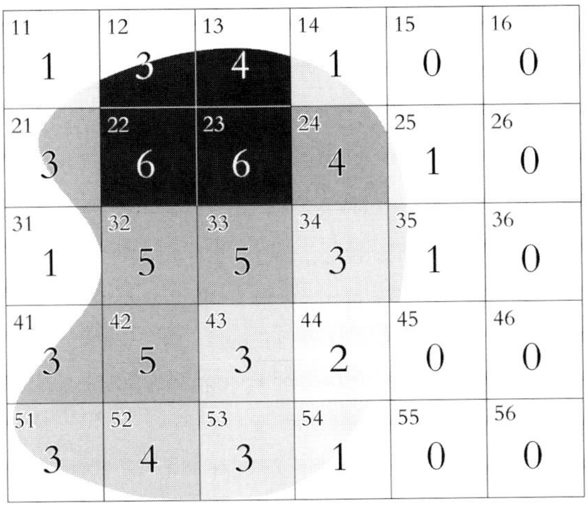

11	12	13	14	15	16
1	3	4	1	0	0
21	22	23	24	25	26
3	6	6	4	1	0
31	32	33	34	35	36
1	5	5	3	1	0
41	42	43	44	45	46
3	5	3	2	0	0
51	52	53	54	55	56
3	4	3	1	0	0

Pixel address	Pixel value
–	–
–	–
25	1
26	0
31	1
32	5
33	5
34	3
35	1
36	0
41	3
42	5
–	–
–	–
–	–

Figure 45. Digital representation of an image. The image is partitioned by an imaginary grid into thousands, or even millions, of tiny, square pixels. Every point on the image is assigned a unique pixel address number, and its shade of gray or color is expressed as the numerical pixel value. An entire image can then be represented completely as a listing of pixel addresses and corresponding pixel values.

shown in figure 46. There, within a light-proof box, the film lies flat on a horizontal glass plate. A laser points at it from above, and a computer-controlled mechanical or electro-optical device deflects and aims the narrow laser beam to successive points on the film. The amount of laser light that gets through any small area of the film is continuously monitored by a photodetector beneath the glass plate.

To begin digitization, the computer partitions the film into an imaginary matrix of square picture elements—whose dimensions are roughly those of the laser beam itself—and assigns a spatial address to each. It then directs the laser beam to the first of these pixels, and the photodetector generates a voltage proportional to the amount of laser light transmitted through that tiny area of film. The signal voltage from the photodetector is measured and electronically digitized—transformed into an ordinary number, expressed in bits and bytes. This number is sent back to the computer, which now knows both the position and the amount of darkening of this small portion of film. The laser beam then proceeds rapidly to the next pixel location, and the photodetector samples the film transparency there, too, and generates the corresponding pixel value, and so on. The two-dimensional matrix of numbers produced in this fashion is called a "bit map." The computer can store—or send to California electronically—the bit map as a long string of pixel addresses and values.

Once in the computer, and perhaps after some digital enhancement, the

A glass thermometer and you, together, nicely illustrate the idea of digitization. The length of the mercury column varies continuously with the temperature but, in sampling it, you read it off as a discrete number to the nearest tenth of a degree. The device that does the same kind of thing with electrical signals is called an analog-to-digital converter (ADC).

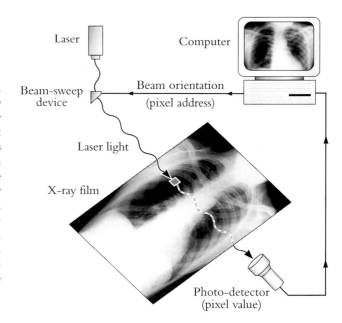

Figure 46. Digitizing an X-ray film. After setting up an imaginary matrix, the computer directs a laser beam from pixel to pixel and, at each stop, a photodetector samples the amount of light passing through the film; the voltage from the photodetector is digitized, or translated into an ordinary number, and entered back into the computer. The image can be recovered, on a video monitor or laser printer, by feeding pixel address and pixel brightness information to the display device.

image can be made to reappear on a display by reversing the digitization process. The computer pulls up all the stored pixel addresses and pixel values for a single image, and places them in proper sequence according to the raster pattern. The digital numeric address of the first pixel is converted into voltages that, for a television monitor, deflect its electron beam so that the point of light on the screen moves to the correct pixel location; the pixel value controls the display brightness (and perhaps color) there. Then on to the second pixel. This happens extraordinarily quickly, of course, but the individual steps are straightforward.

For the film digitizer, the laser-plus-photodetector system scanned a radiograph and generated a signal voltage that was then digitized and sent to a computer. As the following chapters show, other digital imaging systems work much the same way. The types of radiation that interact with the patient's body and then with the detector(s) differ considerably among different imaging modalities, but for all cases the process is basically the same: a detector senses radiation coming from or modified by the body, and produces a corresponding signal voltage. This electrical signal is digitized and sent to a computer, which produces two- or three-dimensional images that reflect the characteristics of the tissues within the region being examined.

Some information is inevitably lost in sampling and digitizing and redisplaying, so the system must be designed to ensure that the image is not so badly degraded that it is no longer useful. Figure 47a, for example, is a typical clinical MRI image produced with a 256 × 256 pixel matrix and 256

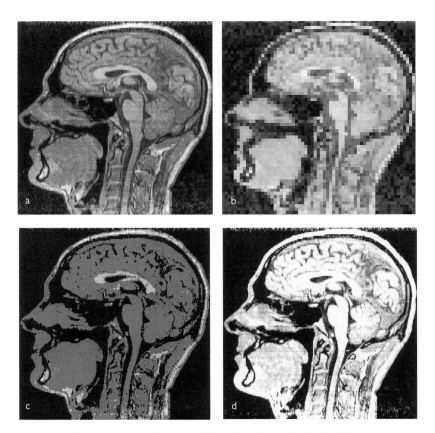

Figure 47. The importance of many small pixels and enough shades of gray.
(a) An MRI image of the head, with a 256 × 256 pixel matrix and 256 shades of gray.
(b) A 64 × 64 image with 256 gray levels. (c) 256 × 256, but with only four levels of
gray. (d) The physician can adjust the windowing, the relationship between the
different shades of gray of the image pixels and (for CT, for example) the different
amounts of X-ray attenuation in the tissue voxels. Although 256 levels of gray scale
are employed here, the image conveys little information because the windowing
chosen is far from optimal. Courtesy of W. S. Kiger III, Massachusetts Institute of
Technology.

shades of gray. Nothing smaller than a pixel can be imaged, so fine features
will be missed if the pixels are too large relative to the entity being viewed,
and too small in number, as in figure 47b. Likewise, even with good resolution, the image will not convey sufficient information unless there are
enough distinct gray levels available (figure 47c). And even with an adequate pixel matrix and gray scale, the image will appear over- or underexposed unless the levels of gray are set so as to span and reflect the proper
range for the tissue characteristic being imaged (figure 47d).

With a matrix two thousand pixels on a side, a digital radiographic image is nearly indistinguishable from an ordinary X-ray film. CT and MRI
enjoy less inherent spatial resolution, by comparison, and often there is
little harm in adopting a coarser pixel matrix, such as 512 × 512, to cover

roughly the same region of the body. Nuclear medicine and ultrasound generally require even less fineness. Fewer pixels (or gray levels) per image means faster image reconstruction and processing, and lower storage and communication costs. Thus, an important objective in designing or purchasing imaging equipment is to create an overall system with more than enough capability to accomplish the requisite clinical tasks, but not much beyond that, to keep the cost down.

X-RAY FILMS WITHOUT FILM: DIGITAL RADIOGRAPHY

I have described how an ordinary X-ray film can be optically scanned for input into a computer. Digital radiology is a technology in which planar X-ray images are obtained without ever being placed on film—a great leap beyond film digitization.

With one common form of digital radiography, an *imaging plate* coated with a photosensitive phosphor replaces the film-screen cassette as the image receptor, as in figure 48. After a normal X-ray exposure, the imaging plate is not developed chemically, like a film. Instead, it is placed inside a light-tight box, and a laser beam of one color of light scans it in a raster pattern while a photodetector continuously monitors how much fluorescent light of a different color is emitted. The brightness of the stimulated light coming from any point on the plate is proportional to the amount of X-ray energy that has passed through the patient and been deposited there. The X-ray image is recovered in the form of the time-varying voltage from the photodetector, somewhat like that from the target of a video camera, and entered into a computer.

Digital radiography offers several benefits. With conventional film X rays, the film has to play two distinct and separate roles. First, it acquires the image; then, after it is developed, it serves as the means of storing and displaying the image. The problem is that exposure conditions that create strong shadows and excellent contrast in the (invisible) X-ray beam emerging from the patient's body are not necessarily the same as those that pro-

Figure 48. Digital radiology. The equipment is like that of film X ray, except that the film cassette is replaced with a photosensitive image plate. This image plate, which has been exposed to X rays, is now being read. It is scanned, in the dark, by a narrow laser beam of some color; the amount of visible fluorescent light of a different color emitted from any point on it is proportional to the amount of X-ray energy deposited there during the exposure.

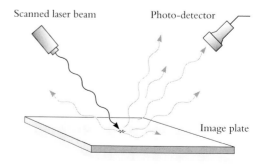

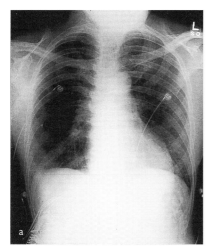 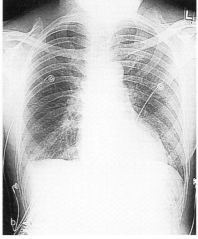

Figure 49. These two images came from the same exposure of an image plate. (a) In one, the image was electronically processed so as to look like a conventional radiograph. (b) The other accentuates sharp edges, such as those of the ribs.

duce high visual quality in the developed film. Exposure conditions that yield strongest X-ray contrast might make areas of the developed film too faint or too dark to be seen clearly—and once a film has been over- or underexposed, little can be done to fix it.

Digital radiography, on the other hand, permits nearly complete decoupling of image formation from image display, so that each can be optimized separately. That is, first the X-ray machine exposure is set at values that give rise to the greatest differences in attenuation of the beam by the various tissues; afterward, and independently, the operator can manipulate the gray scale, activate contrast-enhancement programs or noise-reduction filters, and adjust other display parameters to obtain the most visually effective image (figure 49). This flexibility, along with the general advantages of storing and communicating images digitally from the outset, suggest that despite its greater cost, digital radiography will replace film in many situations. The computer's ability to enhance image contrast and to draw a physician's attention to abnormal image patterns may prove particularly useful where irregularities are most subtle, as in mammography.

Yet an X-ray film system is inexpensive and easy to operate, requires no computers that crash and burn just when they are most needed, and provides a record that can be stored forever on a shelf. So it is probably safe to predict that X-ray films will still be with us, performing many important jobs, for a good while to come.

IN THE EYE OF THE BEHOLDER

The three basic measures of X-ray image quality—resolution, contrast, and noise level—are also relevant for digital images, and we can couch some of these terms in computer-friendly language. Regardless of how a digital image is produced, its information content depends on the fineness of its spatial detail, on the subtlety of the variations in shadings of gray or color that can be distinguished, and on the level of visual noise. The smaller the pixels (and the greater their number, for a given image area), and the more gray levels, and the lower the random fluctuations in the shadings, the more faithfully a digital representation can capture and reproduce clinical reality. At the same time, the computer time and power required to process, ship, and store an image (and hence the cost) rise.

The appearance and the diagnostic worth of an image can improve only so much, though, before the law of diminishing returns sets in. Beyond a certain point, the physician's eye will not be aware of (nor will patients profit from) additional enhancements in spatial resolution or contrast, and further efforts and dollars are largely wasted.

Having considered how digital images are created, stored, and displayed with computers, let's see how and why, in the clinic, they are worth all the effort.

ESSENTIAL ROLES
FOR THE COMPUTER IN IMAGING

Computers play crucial roles in medicine, and nowhere more prominently than in imaging. Although film radiography is still the most common form of imaging, radiologists and other physicians rely more and more on information from computer-based technologies—for several different but interrelated reasons.

Image Reconstruction

Computers, and the digital representation of images, are essential for CT, MRI, and PET. These types of images are not obtained directly, as with X-ray film, but are mathematically constructed out of thousands of separate measurements. Without the ability to orchestrate these measurements and then to manipulate their results numerically, performing millions of computations in a few seconds, such imaging simply would not be possible.

Image Processing

Once it's in digital form, any image can be mathematically massaged to improve its appearance and usefulness. Parts or all of it can be enlarged or reduced, rotated, inverted, stretched, or transformed from a positive image to a negative. The computer can adjust the gray scale, which relates pixel value to brightness, to optimize apparent contrast. It can draw a sharp edge where the shade of gray changes abruptly, so as to increase artificially the sharpness of a border, and thus help the eye to distinguish clinically relevant patterns. Digital filters can reduce some kinds of visual

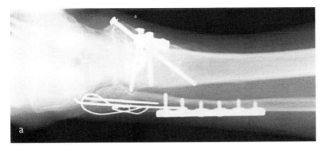

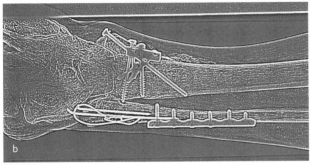

Figure 50. Edge enhancement, one kind of image processing. (a) A digital radiograph that has been deliberately blurred a small amount; you could not visually distinguish it from the original. (b) The computer subtracts the blurred version from the unblurred, pixel by pixel, thereby removing the visual information that is not much affected by the blurring—which, in effect, means the more gradually changing parts of the image, where there are no sharp edges. Left behind is an artificial image in which the edges and sharp features stand out. Courtesy of Agfa, N.V.

noise, compensate for certain inherent inadequacies of the imaging system, and in other ways improve perceived image quality. Such image processing can make the difference between a clinical study that is definitive and one that contributes nothing.

Figure 50 illustrates an interesting and simple way to accentuate sharpness in a digitized radiograph. The idea is something like Michelangelo's explanation of how to carve a *David*—start with a block of marble, and just cut away everything that doesn't look like David. Here, we create a digital copy of our initial image, shown in figure 50a, and deliberately blur it a little; we could replace the value for every pixel, for example, with the average of the values for that pixel and a few of its nearest neighbors. The change is so slight that you probably could not tell the difference by eye, but the image quality has definitely been diminished. Now, by subtracting the blurry copy from what we started out with (that is, by cutting away everything that doesn't look nice and sharp), we end up with the very crisp figure 50b. To make this more visually familiar to the clinician, one can add back some of the original (as was done in figure 10d). The improvement in the sharpened image may not bowl you over, but it might be just enough to reveal some fine features that could make the difference in a diagnosis.

There is always the danger, of course, that such image processing can sometimes lead one to see things that are not really present. A processing program might smooth off a rough surface when it really is rough, for example, or create a sharp edge where there actually should be a gradation.

Image Display

Computers make possible various new kinds of display for images, a flexibility that can enhance both their aesthetic appeal and their clinical usefulness. For example, nuclear medicine and ultrasound commonly use

Figure 51. Three-dimensional display of the skull of a forty-five-year-old citizen of Luxor, Egypt, born 2,200 years ago and now a permanent resident of the Smithsonian Museum. (a) Surface rendering of the skull. (b) The process began with a set of separate, adjacent transverse CT slices. (c) For each, the computer located the bone surfaces, and then stacked the resulting curves in three dimensions. (d) It then tiled over the areas between adjacent contours and added shading. Figure a courtesy of Wayne Olan, George Washington Medical Center, Washington, D.C.

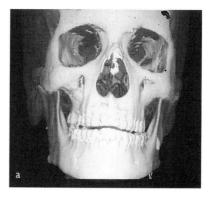

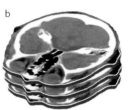 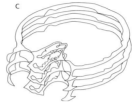 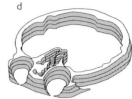

"false colors" that indicate places where interesting things are going on. A PET scan might show areas of unusually high uptake of radionuclide in red, and cooler areas with blue; that may (or may not) be diagnostically helpful. Likewise, some special display programs allow different technologies such as MRI and PET to combine dissimilar kinds of information in a single composite image—a situation in which the diagnostic value of the whole may exceed that of the sum of the parts (see figure 13b).

With volume-imaging modalities, such as multislice CT, MRI, and PET, regions of concern can be shown either in the form of single slices, as in conventional CT, or in three dimensions. The three-dimensional rendering of organs and bones can assist in preoperative planning for neuro-, facial, and orthopedic surgery, and in the planning of radiotherapy cancer treatment. The skull image of figure 51a was built out of a number of separate, adjacent CT cranial slices on a 2,200-year-old patient, until recently a resident of Luxor, Egypt. On every slice, a computer program automatically located each interface between bone and what had been soft tissue, where the X-ray attenuation properties change abruptly, and drew a contour line there (figure 51b). It stacked the curves in three dimensions (figure 51c), and then joined them optically so as to create a smooth cover representing bone surface (figure 51d). Finally, it modulated the shading to give the impression of overlap and depth. It's rather like creating a papier-mâché object by papering over a chicken-wire framework, but here it's all done in the hardware, software, and display monitor of a PC.

One possible next step beyond a three-dimensional image display of a

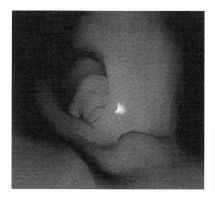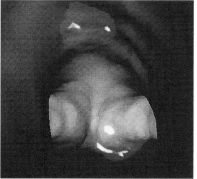

Figure 52 (left). Virtual reality interactive display systems allow the physician to shrink to small size, in effect, and move around within a patient—in this case, along a surface-rendered colon, produced out of a set of MRI scans. Note the polyp, which might give rise to a cancer in the future if not excised, projecting upward from the lower wall in the foreground. Virtual endoscopy is safer for the colon than a standard colonoscopy and a bit less unpleasant for the patient. It can explore far beyond where an endoscope can reach, moreover, and the procedure costs much less. Since colorectal cancer is one of the most common forms of the disease, virtual endoscopy may become an important screening tool for people over age fifty, those at greatest risk. Courtesy of David Vining, Bowman Gray School of Medicine.

Figure 53 (right). Another example of virtual reality: a flight down the trachea, the main air passageway from the mouth and nose, to where it splits into the left and right bronchi that lead to the two lungs. In this image the wall of the trachea has been rendered partially transparent, so that two lymph nodes (lying outside it) have become visible. Courtesy of David Vining, Bowman Gray School of Medicine.

skull is a three-dimensional plastic replication of it. From multislice CT or MRI information, a "fabricator" can generate such an object, one thin layer at a time, from a liquid polymer that hardens when exposed to laser light. Automatic stacking and fusing together of the resulting shaped, solid thin slices can yield a life- (or any other) size model skull that the physician can actually hold—a nearly exact copy of the real thing! (You may have created animals in a similar fashion as a child, gluing together shaped layers of cardboard.)

Virtual reality interactive display systems provide an alternative to solid replications of organs and bones. Virtual endoscopy allows the physician to move around within a three-dimensional block of anatomy, in effect, viewing areas in it from any desired vantage point—along the colon (figure 52), for example, or down the air pathways (figure 53).Until recently the stuff of science fiction, such display systems are coming to play important roles in the planning of surgical cases. They would allow surgeons to employ virtual scalpels to peel away and repair virtual tissue and bone, before actually performing the operation, all the while observing the changes as they occur, and undoing them as needed.

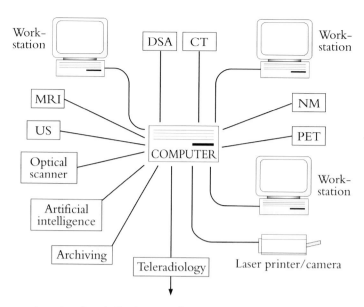

Figure 54. A modern hospital's picture archiving and communications system (PACS), consisting of CT, MRI, nuclear medicine, PET, etc., units, an optical film scanner, artificial intelligence capability, long-distance image communications links (teleradiology), and remote workstations.

Image Archiving and Communications

When in digital form, images from every diagnostic device in a medical center can be entered into a shared computer data base (figure 54). Any study can be stored inexpensively or retrieved almost instantaneously at every work station, integrated with other kinds of information (such as lab reports, electrocardiogram tracings, general medical records, or perhaps even other images), and transmitted through the hospital or across the continent in seconds. Likewise, through *teleradiology*, a digital image produced at an isolated clinic or hospital can be sent by phone or a dedicated channel to a major medical center for examination by specialists. The next case study provides an example of teleradiology. With powerful image archiving and communications capabilities, physicians can obtain and exchange critical information in minutes, rather than days or weeks, and with a wide range of professional colleagues.

Image Analysis and Interpretation

Fascinating, and highly promising, are the computer's growing powers of image analysis and interpretation. Computer-aided diagnosis (CAD) is in its infancy, yet computer-based expert systems, neural networks, and related tools are already playing important new roles in helping physicians make diagnoses. Of particular interest are computer programs adept at pattern recognition. Some have learned to analyze electrocardiograms (which you can think of as one-dimensional images) with success rates comparable to those of cardiologists, and they can do so for hours on end without growing the least bit bleary-eyed. The application of computers to two-dimensional images is far more challenging and will be slower in coming. But the writing is clearly on the wall-mounted, thin-panel liquid crystal display monitor.

Image processing, management, communication, and analysis in the clinic are likely to improve significantly in the near future. The technologies are being developed commercially, and powerful hardware and software tools produced for the military, the intelligence community, the space program, and the basic sciences are being transferred into the medical imaging research laboratories and clinics. It is not obvious where these developments will steer the field, but one thing is certain: the applications of computers in medical imaging will continue to evolve rapidly and to surprise us.

TELERADIOLOGY IN A RURAL SETTING   *CASE STUDY*

Late in the evening, William Herndon, a forty-six-year-old lawyer living near Dead Rock, Nevada, lost control of his DeLorean and crashed into several fence posts. A trucker pulled him from the overturned car and brought him to the Dead Rock Clinic. Mr. Herndon was unconscious and severely battered, but he was breathing regularly and was not hemorrhaging from any external wounds.

The clinic's surgeon, Dr. Julie Nealon, arrived a few minutes before the patient and, immediately after examining him, ordered radiographs. The films revealed several broken ribs and a fractured leg bone, but they were otherwise unremarkable. The spine seemed intact. But Mr. Herndon's blood pressure had begun to fall and his heart rate was increasing. These are signs suggestive of significant blood loss, which could not be explained by the small amount of external bleeding. Clearly more information on the status of the internal organs was needed.

The clinic has a CT machine, and the local doctors are adept at recognizing and diagnosing many common problems with it. But none of them is a radiologist, so for difficult cases they have contracted for teleradiology support from the radiology department of a major West Coast HMO. CT, ultrasound, and occasionally digitally scanned radiographs are sent out for interpretation, the results sometimes arriving back in a matter of minutes.

After discussing the case with the on-call consultant, who was at his home in Berkeley, CT scans of the abdomen were obtained, using radi-

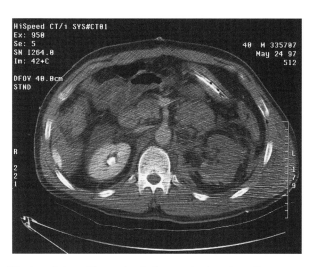

Figure 55. CT teleradiology. The patient's damaged spleen is easily seen on other slices. Here, it appears that while contrast agent is reaching the right kidney (the oval to the left of the vertebral body), none seems to be getting to the left. After receiving the image over the phone lines, the radiologist suggested that this might be caused by the plugging of the renal artery by its lining, torn loose during the accident. If this were true, the kidney would die in a matter of hours without repair of the artery. Despite some loss of image quality during transmission, the scan was adequate to play a defining clinical role, substantially affecting the treatment. Courtesy of John Chotkowski, Associated Radiologists of the Finger Lakes, Elmira, N.Y.

ographic contrast agent. It was immediately clear from a number of the slices that a large amount of blood was collecting in the abdominal cavity; there seemed to be active bleeding from the spleen, which presumably had been lacerated by a fractured rib. But the CT images might also contain subtle signs of other trauma that would be evident only to an experienced radiologist, so Dr. Nealon sent them over the telephone network to the radiologist's home office. Transmission took about two minutes.

The radiologist quickly called back, confirming the damage to the spleen. In addition, he was able to offer an interpretation of something Dr. Nealon had mentioned but, in the heat of trying to keep her critically hurt patient alive, had not dwelled on. Contrast agent was reaching Mr. Herndon's right kidney (the oval to the left of the vertebral body in figure 55— you are looking from his feet toward his head), making it appear pale, with some of it being properly excreted with urine into the renal (kidney) pelvis, the small bright area. Contrast agent (and, by implication, blood) was not getting to the left kidney, however, and it should have been, even if the organ had been injured.

A plausible explanation was that the main artery leading to the left kidney had become obstructed. The kidney is not fixed firmly to the back of the abdominal cavity, and during the rapid deceleration at the moment of the collision, it may have been yanked a considerable distance forward. This could have stretched the renal artery enough to tear its inner lining loose. The dislodged sheet of lining tissue could then have plugged the artery. If this were indeed the case, the kidney, deprived of sufficient blood-borne oxygen, would be irreparably damaged within hours. And although one can live comfortably with a single kidney, it's definitely a better idea to have a spare.

Working on arteries is always a tricky business, but Dr. Nealon had had enough training and experience in vascular surgery to attempt to deal with this problem. Moreover, if her efforts failed, she could always remove the kidney—and if she didn't try, the patient would lose it anyway. Later that night, after she had taken out the spleen and searched carefully for other signs of damage, she performed the necessary repairs on the renal artery which had, indeed, been blocked by its torn inner lining. A week later Mr. Herndon was ready to head home, feeling almost normal, with both kidneys back in working order. Without the teleradiology consultation, he would definitely have lost one of them.

After the accident, Mr. Herndon experienced intermittent sharp pains in his lower back that radiated down his left leg. Dr. Nealon found weakness and decreased sensation in the leg, and somewhat diminished reflexes there. She inspected the X-ray films again, but they revealed no cracks or fractures in the vertebrae, pelvis, or leg bones. She noted that several of the disks, the jelly-filled, Teflonlike pads that serve as cushions between the vertebral bodies, were thinner than others, but this sign of mild degeneration was not surprising for someone the age of her patient. Assuming that the pain might well be attributable to muscle bruising, she addressed this new difficulty with the simplest, most obvious, and least expensive treatment—starting him on anti-inflammatory drugs and keeping him in bed.

When the pain did not subside over a few weeks, even with physiotherapy, she recommended that he go to Las Vegas for an MRI examination of the spine. We shall find him there in chapter 8.

CHAPTER 5

Slices of Life

COMPUTED TOMOGRAPHY (CT)

In film radiography, information from throughout a three-dimensional body is projected onto a two-dimensional plane. In the process, subtle irregularities can become lost in the interplay of image patterns created by overlapping tissue structures. Within the lung, for example, soft-tissue lesions are easily obscured by the strong variations in X-ray beam attenuation caused by the ribs and by the convoluted shapes of the larger air spaces. Likewise for the brain. Nearly all photons entering the head are absorbed or scattered by skull bone, and the tissues within are radiologically nearly homogeneous, anyway, so a film normally reveals little of clinical value.

Digital subtraction angiography can circumvent this problem in one particular kind of study, that of arteries and veins. DSA uses "before" and "after" images to subtract, and thus cancel out, all tissues except the blood vessels that have just been filled with contrast agent opaque to X rays. What remains is the "difference" X-ray image of a three-dimensional network of arteries or veins, with the other, irrelevant (and unchanged) tissues rendered invisible. The problem is that although the approach performs beautifully in the study of blood vessels and in a few other special situations, it isn't much help elsewhere.

Computed tomography (CT) uses a radically different strategy to achieve essentially the same end—the removal of extraneous but visually competing information—and it does so in a way that makes possible the imaging of *any* tissue structure, not just blood vessels. The resulting ability to obtain a clean, cross-sectional view of the body has had an impact on medicine that has been nothing short of revolutionary.

ON THE DENSITY OF LUNG, THE PREDICTION OF AVALANCHES, AND THE FIRST CT SCANNER

In 1955, Allan Cormack, a South African educated at Cambridge University, found himself back at the University of Cape Town, lecturing on nuclear physics and spending one and a half days a week in Groote Schuur Hospital worrying about people's lungs.

The hospital physicist overseeing the use of radioactive materials at Groote Schuur had just resigned; Cormack, the only person in Cape Town qualified to fill in, agreed to help out until a permanent replacement could be found. Cormack's new duties included supervising the planning of radiation therapy treatments for cancer patients. The objective of radiotherapy, as noted in chapter 3, is to kill all the cells of a tumor with ionizing radiation without causing excessive harm to any nearby critical organs in the process. A good treatment plan shows how to aim several high-energy X- or gamma-ray beams into the patient so that their crossfire region fully covers the tumor area, while much lower doses end up in the surrounding healthy tissues. If the tissues within a body were completely homogeneous, like water in a plastic bag, then treatment planning would be easy once the tumor was localized. But the differences in density and chemical makeup between, say, the lungs and bones of a real patient radically affect the patterns of radiation dose deposition, and should be taken into account. As of 1955, however, no one had yet figured out an effective way to do that.

Cormack found this problem interesting, obviously extremely important, little explored, and quite possibly solvable—a physicist's dream! The critical element, he saw, would be an image that mapped out, point by point within the patient, how readily the various tissues remove X-ray energy from a beam. And the only way to produce this map, in practice, would be from measurements made outside the body. But if such images could be produced, Cormack realized, they might well have significant diagnostic applications far beyond radiotherapy treatment planning.

Over the next few years, he devised a process for generating his tissue map. First, he would acquire a great deal of data on the amounts of energy removed as an X-ray beam systematically cut numerous different specific paths through a patient. This involved pointing narrow beams at the body from various directions and measuring the reduction in their intensities as they emerged from the far side. Then he would carry out a complex mathematical procedure he had devised to translate the set of measurements of beam attenuation, just obtained, into the desired image.

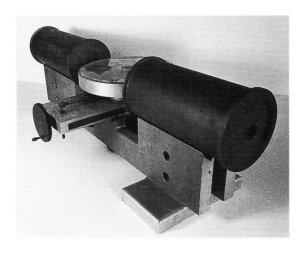

Figure 56. Allan Cormack built this device in 1963 for about $100 and produced the first X-ray computed tomography images with it. Courtesy of Allan Cormack.

Cormack assembled a simple tabletop apparatus in 1963 to test his approach (figure 56). His first "patient" was a block of plastic containing two aluminum discs (representing tumors in brain), surrounded by an aluminum ring skull. The results clearly revealed the details of his patient's construction—he had, indeed, envisaged and built the first working CT device. Cormack has described the frenzy of enthusiasm that ensued: "Publication took place in 1963 and 1964. There was virtually no response. The most interesting request for a reprint came from the Swiss Center for Avalanche Research. The method would work for deposits of snow on mountains if one could get either the detector or the source [of radiation] into the mountain under the snow!"[1]

Eventually Cormack's teaching and nuclear physics research pulled him away from medical work, and he gave his map of the tissues little further thought until the early 1970s.

At the 1972 Annual Congress of the British Institute of Radiology, the English firm EMI, Ltd., stunned the radiological community with the unveiling of a novel clinical imaging technology, computed tomography. The EMI device came into being primarily through the efforts of Godfrey Hounsfield, who was unaware of Cormack's earlier work. For their respective contributions to this work, Hounsfield and Cormack shared the 1979 Nobel prize for physiology or medicine.

In retrospect, there seems to be a certain inevitability to the invention of computed tomography. As is often the case in science, researchers were working on closely related projects, albeit in fields as seemingly disparate as radio astronomy, electron microscopy, nuclear medicine, and the prediction of avalanches—and some were on paths that might well have converged on CT itself. If Cormack had not thought the process through and produced a bench-scale device, and if Hounsfield had not put all the pieces

Also deserving of a note of appreciation are John, Paul, George, and Ringo; it was largely through the enormous influx of cash from the Beatles' recordings that EMI (Electrical and Musical Industries), Ltd., was able to support the development of Hounsfield's scanner.

together and built a commercial machine in the late 1960s, in all likelihood someone else would have done so soon thereafter. This is not to detract from Cormack's and Hounsfield's splendid achievements—but given the growing access to computers and the rapidly expanding interest in the field of digital imaging technology, CT was clearly a marvelous idea whose time had come.

CASE STUDY   A CT EXAM THAT DOES *NOT* REVEAL A STROKE

Frank Pulank, a seventy-year-old musician, has brought to thousands of people the joys of Beethoven, Bach, and Mozart. As his northern Vermont community grew from an isolated farming village into an exurb of Burlington, he gave performances each year in churches, school auditoriums, and civic centers throughout the region. And by the time he retired last year, he had taught countless grade- and high-school students to play piano and band instruments.

One morning a month ago, he awoke with considerable numbness in his left arm and leg, and he was unable to move either. Unfortunately, his wife was visiting her sister and did not find him until noon, still lying in bed and very disoriented and confused—he hadn't even thought to use the phone for help. His wife called an ambulance, and Dr. Ravelle, a grand-nephew, met them at the emergency room.

Mr. Pulank has had a blood pressure problem for years, but he has taken his medication erratically. In examining him, Dr. Ravelle found his blood pressure to be at its usual high level. Mr. Pulank couldn't remember the names of the days of the week or—of much greater concern to him—the lovely melodies that normally wove through his thoughts. Also, his speech was slurred and he was unable to carry out some simple commands. His left arm and leg were insensitive to pinpricks and appeared paralyzed. It was clear that Mr. Pulank had suffered a stroke, and that his condition was serious.

There are two general types of stroke, hemorrhagic and ischemic, and either kind can range in severity from minor to fatal. In a hemorrhagic stroke, generally the more serious kind, a weakened spot in the wall of a blood vessel in the brain balloons outward and eventually ruptures, flooding the area with blood. Pressure builds up locally because more blood enters the flooded region than exits from it, and because the irritated brain tissue itself becomes inflamed and swollen. Local compression of brain tissue prevents fresh, oxygen-rich blood from reaching the afflicted area and slowly strangles it. An ischemic stroke, by contrast, involves a partial or complete blockage of a cerebral blood vessel. This plugging might be

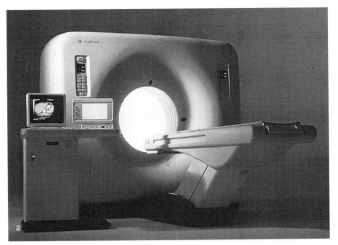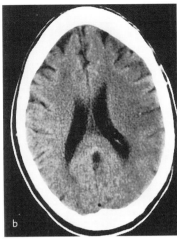

Figure 57. Computed tomography. (a) A modern CT machine. (b) The scans of this stroke patient all appeared normal, even with contrast agent. Figure a courtesy of General Electric Medical Systems.

caused by a blood clot originating in the heart or elsewhere. Or, in a person with arteriosclerosis (hardening of the arteries), a piece of plaque (a small plate or pebble of cholesterol) may break loose from inside the aorta, or perhaps from an artery of the neck, and lodge in a narrower stretch of blood vessel of the brain. This, too, can prevent adequate oxygenation of its tissues.

Mr. Pulank was sent immediately for a CT scan which, it was hoped, would allow an assessment of the amount and location of brain tissue affected. That knowledge, in turn, would help in guiding treatment and making a prognosis. And providing the right treatment early could substantially improve his odds for recovery, or at least help to contain the damage.

In the CT suite, Mr. Pulank lay on his back on the table of the CT machine, with the top of his head positioned just inside the hole of the large, doughnut-shaped gantry (figure 57a). An intravenous (IV) catheter was inserted into a vein of his arm for the subsequent injection of iodine-based contrast agent, if needed.

The study began as the table advanced slowly through the gantry aperture. The patient seemed to understand the technician's repeated instructions, relayed into the examination room by intercom, to take a deep breath and hold still. The emergence of his head from the far side of the aperture marked the completion of the first phase of the examination, and a series of clear CT images appeared on a TV monitor. Each one shows a transverse slice through the head, a few millimeters thick (figure 57b). The dense bone of the skull comes out white, and the various brain tissues emerge in shades of gray. The normal convolutions of the brain are visible at its surface, just inside the skull. The salt-water-like cerebrospinal fluid that bathes the brain looks black.

This first set of images gave no indication of a stroke. Mr. Pulank was repositioned, some radiographic contrast agent (the same kind of iodine-based material as is used in conventional radiography) was injected through the IV tube, and the entire procedure was repeated. In healthy brain tissue, contrast material would be swept quickly in and out as the blood passes through its vessels. When brain material has suffered certain kinds of trauma, however, some of the entering contrast material will seep out of the arteries and veins and remain behind—indicating a breach in the "blood-brain barrier." But despite Mr. Pulank's obvious symptoms, this study proved negative as well. Radiologically, the brain looked normal.

The radiologist suggested that because the stroke was recent, its effects might not yet be far enough advanced to show up on CT. A magnetic resonance imaging study, he knew, is more sensitive to certain subtle aspects of tissue physiology than CT, and might be more revealing. So we shall return to Mr. Pulank in chapter 8, in the MRI department.

HOW CT "SEES"

Imagine that you can, without causing too much disruption, temporarily pluck a pancake-thin cross-sectional slice from a patient's body for radiographic study (figure 58). You place the slice on a cassette, and briefly turn on an overhead X-ray tube. Anywhere in the resulting image, the darkness of the developed film is determined by, and reflects, the attenuation properties of the little piece of tissue that was lying directly above it. The contrast among soft tissues would be good enough for you to distinguish many of the organs from one another (unlike the contrast in an ordinary radiograph), the resolution would be fine, and noise would be low.

Where there is bone, few X rays get through, and the film ends up pale and translucent, with little metallic silver in it—and the opposite occurs where there is soft tissue.

For various technical and legal / ethical reasons, this approach is unlikely to find widespread clinical acceptance. Fortunately there is a back door to the same place: computed tomography. A CT picture of our slice, back in the intact patient, as with figure 57b, would look almost exactly like what we saw with figure 58. It, too, shows how the attenuation of X rays by tissues varies from point to point within the slice.

The main difference between the two views is not what we see, but rather how the image is produced. Since shooting directly down through the slice of interest is not an option, CT takes an indirect approach. It first

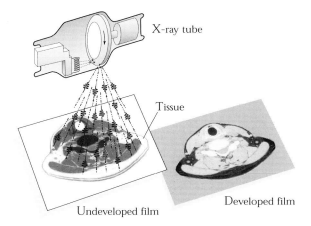

X-ray tube

Tissue

Undeveloped film

Developed film

Figure 58. The hypothetical situation in which we carry out a normal X-ray film examination of a pancake-thin, transverse slice of tissue carved out of a patient. CT will produce a nearly identical image (but with less of the mess). To do so, though, it has to rely on numerous attenuation measurements, with beams passing through the patient from all sides.

makes thousands of X-ray transmission measurement studies of the region, with the X-ray tube and X-ray detector(s) situated outside the body and facing one another. Its computer then performs a tremendous number of sophisticated computations to calculate what the inside of the body must be like so as to yield this particular measured set of transmission data.

Suppose a father has found his two-year-old taking small objects from his desk and perhaps swallowing them. A radiologist takes a film of the child from the front, which reveals a solid ellipse and, apparently, two loops of wire, but nothing can be identified with certainty. She then films the child from the side, hoping she'll be able to make sense of the two films together (figure 59). What entities, and in what configuration, could possibly give rise to this particular pair of radiographs? With a fair degree of certainty, she deduces that the child swallowed one small coin and two paper clips. Images obtained from several more angles could support this hy-

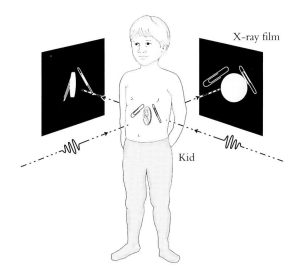

X-ray film

Kid

Figure 59. Although a radiograph of a child's stomach taken from any single angle may not reveal much with certainty, a few pictures together may allow you to determine what he has eaten.

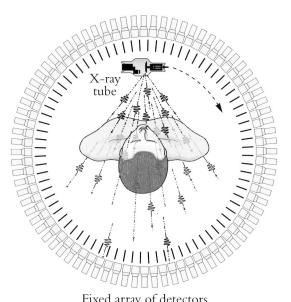

X-ray
tube

Figure 60. With this fourth-generation scanner, the X-ray fan beam is wide enough to cut completely across the patient from any angle, but the irradiated slice is still only a few millimeters thick. The X-ray tube moves along a circle, always pointing inward, and the intensity of beam transmitted through the patient is sensed by a fixed ring of hundreds or thousands of detectors.

Fixed array of detectors

pothesis, whereas an ingested object of more complicated form or internal structure might require even more views. The essential point is this: by thinking properly about, and integrating, pieces of two-dimensional information obtained from several perspectives, one can construct, or at least imagine, a three-dimensional picture that is much, much more revealing than what can be learned from any single view alone.

That, in essence, is how CT works. It creates, digitizes, and stores in a computer the X-ray shadows from a large number (typically 700 to 1,500) of different perspectives. Its computer then works backward from the data just obtained to "reconstruct" mathematically the spatial distribution within the body of the materials (or, more precisely, the spatial distribution of the X-ray attenuation properties of the materials) responsible for this particular set of 700 to 1,500 images.

Some specialized imaging devices, which can perform both fluoroscopy and CT for radiotherapy treatment planning, operate exactly as discussed in the paper clip example, with the beam that emerges from the patient exposing an image intensifier and video camera. But most of what reaches the image intensifier is scatter radiation, and this can greatly reduce image quality. That is why film radiography employs antiscatter grids. Normal diagnostic CT has adopted a different trick to eliminate scatter: instead of irradiating a large, rectangular block of tissue, as with fluoroscopy or film, only a thin, transverse slice of tissue is exposed in the first place. That is, the housing that supports the X-ray tube has a narrow, slit-shaped X-ray window that lets out only a "fan"

Recall that you can reduce scatter degradation in film radiography also by choosing a small X-ray beam size. That's exactly what we're going to do here.

beam, wider than a person but only a few millimeters high (figure 60). An encircling ring of hundreds or thousands of small, independent radiation detectors is able to sense how much radiant energy in any part of that fan beam makes it through and emerges from the far side of the patient. Because the slice is so thin, little scatter radiation is produced within the patient, and nearly all that is generated scatters randomly away from the plane of the detectors.

Thus CT chops the body into thin, transverse slices of anatomy, in effect, and views each one separately from the side, from multiple angles, with X rays. In so doing, it manages to create slice-images of superb clarity and tissue contrast. The necessary mathematical manipulations are complex, and must be carried out on a fast computer, but the general concept is simple.

THE NUTS AND BOLTS OF A CT SCANNER

The first commercial CT scanner was designed by Hounsfield to image the head. The X-ray tube and housing window produced a square (rather than fan) beam of very small cross-sectional area, several millimeters on a side, and it was monitored by a single radiation detector. The tube and detector were mounted rigidly on opposite ends of a supporting gantry, with their positions fixed relative to one another. The beam always pointed directly into the detector, with the patient in between, but the tube and detector, in tandem, could undergo both linear and rotational motion relative to the patient.

To generate X-ray attenuation data, the tube and detector were together swept sideways across the patient's head, as in figure 61, so that the narrow beam cut across (and irradiated only) a pancakelike slice of brain tissue a few millimeters thick. During the sweep, the detector made 160 distinct measurements of beam transmission through the head. Then the gantry was rotated through 1 degree about the patient. The beam and detector moved laterally again (slicing along the same plane of tissue as before, but from a slightly different angle), and 160 new measurements were made. This sweep-then-rotate procedure was repeated 180 times, once per degree, until the gantry had swung halfway around the patient. The system thus made $180 \times 160 = 28{,}800$ separate X-ray transmission measurements for a single thin slice of tissue.

A computer unraveled all the resulting data by means of a reconstruction computation and calculated the relative amount of X-ray attenuation at each of thousands of points within the slice. It then displayed these values on a monitor, with light and dark shades corresponding, respectively, to relatively high and low amounts of local attenuation. Because the rate

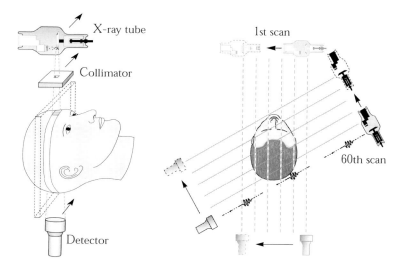

Figure 61. In Hounsfield's first CT scanner, the X-ray tube and the single detector moved in tandem laterally across the patient, and the narrow X-ray beam cut out a thin transverse slice. The gantry was then rotated through a small angle and the procedure repeated.

of X-ray attenuation at a given point depends on the type of tissue at that point, the process generated a clinically useful map of human anatomy within the slice.

Since Hounsfield's day, CT image quality has improved phenomenally, and the time required to produce a slice image has dropped to practically nothing. Modern machines have eliminated the need for the slow linear motions of the X-ray tube and radiation detectors across the patient. The X-ray tube of a fourth-generation scanner, for example, rapidly circles the patient, with a fan beam always pointing inward, toward the center, as shown in figure 60. The transmitted beam is sampled by a ring of many small, closely spaced, immobile detectors. In a fifth-generation machine, not even the X-ray tube moves, and it can produce a picture in a few hundredths of a second. This is fast enough to freeze the motions of the heart.

As with radiography and fluoroscopy, three desirable attributes of CT images are strong tissue contrast, low noise, and fine resolution. CT provides a contrast capability that is quite high, compared with standard film radiography. A 0.5 percent difference in attenuation rate between tissues is typically detectable by CT—ten times better than with a radiographic film. On the other hand, the best resolution achievable is something like a third of a millimeter in the body, ten or more times poorer than with film. That is why one selects CT when good contrast among soft tissues is important but minute detail is not. The level of visual noise that shows up

Some modern scanners take data continuously as the patient table glides slowly but smoothly through the gantry aperture. The X-ray beam cuts out a multiturn helical pattern within the body, with adjacent loops of the helix only millimeters apart, and the computer then adjusts the images to end up with the usual set of parallel transverse slices. Helical scanning is very fast, making possible novel clinical applications.

depends on several factors, such as the slice thickness chosen (typically, a few millimeters), the resolution required, and the dose imparted to the patient; these are generally balanced against one another in such a way that noise is not a limiting problem.

Finally, the dose throughout the exposed volume is several rem. Although that is not excessive, it *is* considerably greater than one generally finds with most other imaging techniques. That, and the relatively high cost, are why physicians do not prescribe CT studies unless there is a good medical reason to do so.

CT CONSTRUCTS A MAP OF X-RAY ATTENUATION

Let us return to the question of what it is, exactly, that a CT image reveals. The tendency of a tissue (or other material) to remove X-ray energy from a beam is quantified in terms of the attenuation coefficient (also called the attenuation rate, and usually represented by μ, the Greek letter mu). This coefficient may be defined as the spatial rate of attenuation that the beam experiences in traversing a thin slice of material. The greater the value of μ for a tissue, the more rapidly the beam is absorbed or scattered in it.

The discussion in chapter 2 of the absorption and scattering of X-ray photons by matter indicated that the value of μ for a piece of tissue depends on its density and effective atomic number (as well as on the average photon energy for the beam). Thus, by mapping out spatial variations in the attenuation coefficient within each slice, resulting from differences in tissue density and chemical makeup, CT provides an image of the anatomy. That is exactly what an ordinary radiograph does, of course, only not slice by slice.

Imagine a transverse slice of a human body that is partitioned with an imaginary grid into a matrix of *voxels,* or tiny blocks of tissue, each about a millimeter on a side and as tall as the slice is thick. The grid size is commonly expressed in terms of the number of voxels in each dimension—a 512×512 matrix, for example, contains about a quarter million of them.

As suggested by figure 62, image reconstruction involves back-calculating, from the results of thousands of radiation transmission measurements on a slice of tissue, the relative amount of attenuation (i.e., the value of μ) occurring separately at every voxel within it. The computed map of the attenuation rates is then displayed as a mosaic of pixels of various shades of gray, usually with a single pixel in the image corresponding to each voxel in the tissue slice.

In summary: The CT image of a tissue slice is a voxel-by-voxel pixel-map of the values of the tissue X-ray attenuation coefficient throughout it.

If the intensity of a particular X-ray beam is diminished by 2.5 percent in passing through 0.1 centimeter (1 mm) of a certain tissue, for example, then the attenuation coefficient there, μ, has the value (0.025 / 0.1 cm) = 0.25 per cm.

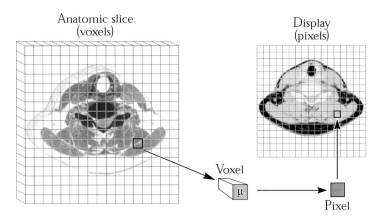

Anatomic slice
(voxels)

Display
(pixels)

Voxel

μ

Pixel

Figure 62. CT image reconstruction refers to the process by which a computer transforms a set of transmission measurements into a two-dimensional array of voxel attenuation-rate values; these, in turn, can subsequently be displayed as a corresponding matrix of pixels of various shades of gray or color on a video monitor. Windowing of the gray scale helps to optimize image quality (see figure 47d).

THE STANDARD RECONSTRUCTION ALGORITHM

Several mathematical reconstruction methods have been devised for translating a set of attenuation measurements into a pixel map. Perhaps the easiest to visualize is known as the algebraic reconstruction technique (ART), illustrated in figure 63. Suppose that a hypothetical patient consists of only four voxels, with attenuation coefficients labeled as in figure 63a. Horizontal transmission measurements are made, and the attenuation by the entire lower and upper rows of voxels are found to be 4 and 3, say, in the appropriate units. Likewise, vertical measurements yield 5 and 2 units of attenuation for the two columns. Finally, the diagonals give 1 and 6. Computer programs that have been available for years can rapidly determine that the only possible set of values for the attenuation coefficients of our four voxels are the ones displayed in the pixel map of figure 63b—which, in fact, defines the CT image for our patient. This reconstruction method is not optimal, but it does work. It was hoped that ART could be speeded up considerably by coupling it with a powerful mathematical technique known as the Fast Fourier Algorithm (FFA), which has been employed successfully with other approaches to reconstruction, but the work was severely hampered by lack of a suitable acronym.

The only reconstruction technique currently used in commercial CT machines is filtered back-projection (which *does* use the FFA). The math-

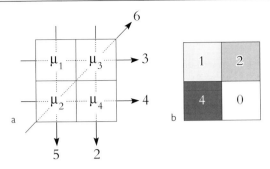

Figure 63. Algebraic reconstruction technique. (a) The four voxels of our patient, and the amounts of attenuation measured. (b) The only configuration of voxel attenuation values consistent with the measurements.

ematical details are involved, but the basic idea is straightforward. Let us examine the simplest of all possible patients, a humanlike test "phantom" that is transparent to X rays everywhere except at one bone sliver (figure 64). Our objective is to find and display the position of the single high-density voxel.

It is easiest to talk about a scanner of Hounsfield's original design, with a very narrow X-ray beam, one voxel wide. Typically, 180 different beam angles are required to generate an image, but for locating our single opaque voxel, two will suffice.

We start by orienting the X-ray beam horizontally and positioning it just below the bottom of the phantom, as in figure 64a. At the same time, we establish a corresponding pixel coordinate system on the display monitor. With this first beam angle, we repeatedly carry out a three-step procedure:

1. Measure the attenuation by the phantom of the narrow X-ray beam;

2. Lay down (back-project) a narrow stripe, one pixel wide, at the corresponding level on the display. The brightness of the stripe shown on the monitor is to be proportional to the amount of attenuation of the X-ray beam along this path through the phantom, as determined in step 1. Where there is no attenuation, the stripe is made transparent; and

3. Move the X-ray beam one voxel-width upward, and the line on the display one pixel up, and return to step 1.

In other words, carry out the attenuation measurement and back-project, in the first and second steps; shift one voxel position upward in

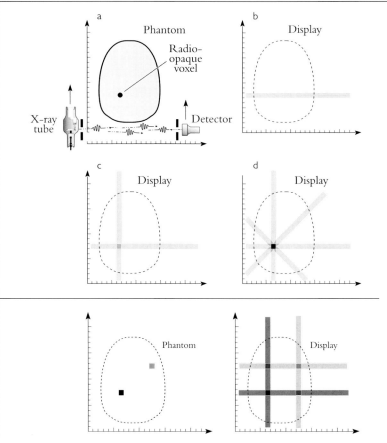

Figure 64 (top). Back-projection image reconstruction. (a) This phantom is transparent to X rays at all voxels but one, which contains a piece of bone. The narrow, horizontally oriented X-ray beam and the detector are stepped upward together and, along the way, locate the level of the opaque voxel. (b) The system displays a horizontal stripe on the monitor at the corresponding level. (c) The procedure is repeated, but with a vertically oriented beam moving left to right. The crossing of the two stripes on the display identifies the opaque voxel. (d) With more measurement angles, the individual stripes become less noticeable.

Figure 65(bottom). With two opaque voxels, two gantry angles are not suffcient.

the phantom, and one pixel up on the display, and then start the procedure over again. For this first (horizontal) orientation of the X-ray beam, repeat the three-step process 160 times, enough to cover the entire phantom (along with some empty space at the bottom and top). With our example of the single opaque voxel, the profile of beam attenuation across the phantom will be reflected on the display as a single, narrow stripe (figure 64b).

Now rotate the X-ray beam and the display line through an appropriate angle, 90 degrees for this exercise, and walk through the whole process again—this time progressing from left to right. A new (vertical) stripe will eventually appear on the display, intersecting the horizontal stripe at the pixel in the image that corresponds to the opaque voxel in the phantom (figure 64c). (The computer doesn't actually create an image one stripe at a time, but its memory does keep track of where the stripes would be, and displays on a video monitor the overall image they collectively generate.) Two X-ray beam alignments happen to be enough to locate our target unambiguously. The pixel corresponding to the highly attenuating voxel is twice as bright as elsewhere along the individual back-projection slices, and back-projecting at many more gantry angles enhances that distinction (figure 64d).

But one pixel does not an image make. Let's try this again on a considerably more challenging phantom with *two* partially opaque voxels, the rate of attenuation in one of them being twice that in the other. Back-projections obtained from two profiles (as before) intersect at four places (figure 65), and it is not immediately obvious which two of them are "real." A third scan resolves the issue, however, since back-projections from the three angles will all overlap at only two places. Expansion of this argument leads to the conclusion that enough back-projection profiles can generate a map of local X-ray attenuation for any real slice of tissues.

Image quality can be significantly enhanced by incorporating a suitable mathematical filter into the back-projection calculation. This causes any single stripe in the image to be replaced with a narrow bundle of several adjacent stripes that have different, cleverly selected levels of darkness. Some of them are even of negative brightness, in the sense that they subtract from other bundles, coming in at other angles, wherever they may overlap. Adding a good filter to back-projection renders the stripes vanishingly faint everywhere except where they intersect. This business may sound complicated, but the whole filtered back-projection image reconstruction process can be accomplished with surprisingly few lines of computer code.

AN OVARIAN TUMOR

Pam Heisenger, who emigrated to upstate New York with her German parents at the age of eight, is a fifty-year-old physics teacher in a community college. She is a slender woman who eats intelligently, exercises daily, consumes alcohol sparingly, smokes not at all, and has a history of good health. Her marriage of thirty years to a lawyer with a nonprofit environmental advocacy group is childless, loving, and largely stress-free.

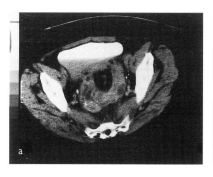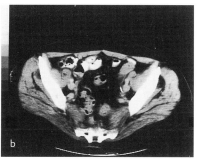

Figure 66. CT studies of a patient with an ovarian tumor. (a) Prior to surgery and chemotherapy, much of the space directly in front of the vertebral body is filled with tumor. (b) The post-treatment images show no evidence of disease.

Recently, Dr. Heisenger felt a vague lower abdominal discomfort and swelling, and found that she had gained five pounds. This combination prompted her to visit her internist. The physical examination revealed three notable abnormalities. During percussion of her abdomen, a region of dull sound shifted when she rolled from her back to her left side, indicating the presence of fluid within. Also of serious concern was the pelvic examination: between his hands, one on the abdomen and the other within the vagina, her physician could feel a hard, fixed mass about the size of a softball. This might be a cyst or benign growth or, of much greater significance, a tumor of the ovary, uterus, or colon. Finally, the results of a blood test revealed, two days later, an elevated level of the protein CA125, which was strongly suggestive of an ovarian malignancy.

This diagnosis was confirmed with a CT study. Figure 66a shows a transverse slice of Dr. Heisenger's pelvis, just below the navel, as she lies on her back. Visible at the top of the scan is her bladder, containing urine and contrast material. The bright regions below the bladder on the left and right are slices through the pelvic bone. At the very bottom of the scan is one of the vertebral bodies of her backbone. In the middle of these landmarks is a large tumor, which originated within one of the ovaries but now extends beyond it. The mass appears mostly solid, but it has become so large that it has outgrown its blood supply, and its center has died and liquefied. Fortunately, none of the forty-four CT slices taken indicated any evidence that the cancer extended beyond the pelvis, to nearby lymph nodes, or to the liver in particular.

Dr. Heisenger underwent ovarian cancer surgery for the removal of the tumor and of the female reproductive organs: both of her ovaries were excised, along with the fatty material surrounding them, as were her fallopian tubes and her uterus, which are paths that commonly allow spread of the disease. The bulk tumor and a margin of healthy tissue around it were taken out, but at the time the surgeon could not be absolutely certain that he had excised 100 percent of the cancerous tissue. Subsequent examination by a pathologist showed no tendrils of malignant tissues extending out of the removed mass—a good sign. Two weeks later, her CA125 level had fallen, but not to zero, suggesting the possibility of residual disease somewhere in her body.

After her incisions had healed sufficiently, Dr. Heisenger began a course of chemotherapy, in an attempt to destroy any cancer cells that might have escaped the surgery. She completed six cycles of treatment, one per month. For each, she returned to the hospital as an outpatient on three consecutive days, and received medication intravenously for two hours. She lost all her hair temporarily and, for about five days after each treatment, she felt somewhat nauseated and experienced minor hot flashes. Chemotherapy has been improving a good deal recently, though, and she did not have to endure the wrenching side effects that some of her friends struggled through in the past. The process was unpleasant, but Dr. Heisenger believed that the increased chances of a full recovery were well worth the price.

A recent CT scan of the pelvis indicates that Dr. Heisenger may have had a complete response to surgery and chemotherapy (figure 66b). Her most recent CA125 level provides further evidence of the absence of disease. Although 75 percent of women with advanced ovarian cancer respond at least partially to treatment, only 20 percent have a total and permanent recovery. Dr. Heisenger's CT scans and CA125 studies suggest that she may be among the fortunate ones.

When cancer drugs were new, chemotherapy commonly involved repeatedly administering a single chemical agent at a high dose level. Such an agent is a real poison, but one designed to do considerably more harm to cancer cells than to healthy tissues. Unfortunately, its selectivity is not perfect, and patients often experienced severe toxic reactions— like an extreme case of food poisoning, and sometimes worse. Currently, however, some treatments involve combinations of several agents, each given in a lower dose. Together, the ingredients have enough potency to kill tumor cells, but each separately affects the patient in a different way. Thus, the patient feels a number of dissimilar, milder side effects and suffers much less than with the older, single-agent treatment.

6

Like Embers in the Dark

NUCLEAR MEDICINE

Let us return for a moment to the months immediately following Roentgen's momentous discovery. No one had any idea what his strange X rays really were—particles of some sort, perhaps, or an unusual form of ordinary light?—or how they came into being. Many of the world's leading scientists naturally turned their attention to this puzzle. And in so doing, one of them, Henri Becquerel, stumbled on an equally bizarre new phenomenon, radioactivity, which has had an even more profound impact on world affairs than X rays have. He did so by coming from a good family and following a bad hunch.

HENRI BECQUEREL, URANIUM, AND PARIS IN THE SPRINGTIME

Becquerel was the third in a direct line of four generations of outstanding physicists. Henri's grandfather, Antoine Cesar Becquerel, had graduated as an officer from the prestigious École Polytechnique (France's equivalent of MIT and West Point rolled into one) in time to serve under Napoleon between 1810 and 1812. Severely wounded and told he had but a short while to live, Antoine Cesar resigned from the army, got a second opinion, and began a long and brilliant academic career in science. Among his primary interests was luminescence, and he was the first to publish the optical spectra of phosphorescent materials. For these and other efforts, a chair in physics was created for him at the Museum of Natural History in Paris. He published 529 research papers, was appointed director of the museum, and lived to see ninety.

Antoine Cesar's third son, Alexandre Edmond, assisted with his father's experiments as a youngster, also studied at the École Polytechnique, became one of the world's leading authorities on luminescence, and succeeded his father as professor of physics at the museum. One of his findings, that some salts of uranium (an element discovered in 1789) are strongly phosphorescent, would later be of great importance to the work of his own second son, Henri.

Henri Becquerel, the central character of our story, followed in the family tradition and devoted much of his life to the study of luminescent materials. By the time of Roentgen's announced discovery, he had, at the age of forty-three, succeeded *his* father as professor of physics at the museum. (And Henri's only child, Jean, would eventually become the fourth in a line of Becquerels holding that position for 110 years consecutively.)

Henri was intrigued by X rays, like everyone else, and his fascination became all the more intense when he learned of one particular observation by Roentgen: X rays seemed to emanate primarily from the glowing spot on the wall of the vacuum tube where cathode rays appeared to be striking, that is, from a part of the glass that seemed to display fluorescence. Might it be, he reasoned, that whatever causes fluorescence in *any* material will also give rise to Roentgen's rays as well, secondarily, and that the phenomenon had simply never been noticed before? To test this hypothesis, he wrapped a photographic plate in thick black paper, put it in direct sunlight, and placed a piece of phosphorescent material on top. If he were correct, the sun should stimulate the phosphorescent material to emit X rays (as well as light), and the plate would be exposed and darkened even though no light could strike it directly.

His initial negative results did not deter him. He believed that all he needed was a luminescent material that emitted X rays with sufficient intensity. "I had great hopes," he later recalled, "for experimentation with the uranium salts, the fluorescence of which I had studied on an earlier occasion, following the work of my father."[1] Putting a covered photographic plate in the sun and placing a sample of uranyl potassium sulfate on it, he found that the portion of the plate where the sample had been became darkened, exactly as expected. He conveyed this finding to the French Academy of Science on February 24, 1896.

Henri intended to repeat and expand on this experiment right away. He prepared and wrapped a fresh photographic plate but, when the weather in Paris took a turn for the worse, he stuck it in a dark drawer with, as it happened, a sample of the uranium salt resting on it. A few days later, for reasons that remain unclear, he removed the plate and developed it: "Since the sun did not show itself again for several days, I developed the photographic plates on the first of March, expecting to find the images very

A luminescent material emits light of a specific color when stimulated by light of another color, say, or by X rays or electrons. If the emission ceases abruptly when the stimulus is turned off, the substance is said to be fluorescent; otherwise, it is phosphorescent. Emission of light by an object raised to high temperature, such as the filament of an incandescent bulb, occurs by way of a fundamentally different physical process and is not considered to be luminescence.

feeble. On the contrary, the silhouettes appeared with great intensity. I thought at once that the action might be able to go on in the dark."[2]

Becquerel's discovery of radioactivity, and the subsequent isolation of the radioactive elements polonium and radium by Marie Curie and her coworkers, aroused little of the excitement that surrounded X rays. Early applications were few and limited in scope. In medicine, radium-filled hollow needles could be inserted into certain inoperable tumors, with some degree of therapeutic success. And a mixture of fluorescent materials and radium would glow continuously, which made possible luminous meter dials that would remain visible in the dark. There were a few other uses, but that was about it.

Then suddenly in the late 1930s, a discovery about radioactive materials seized and riveted the attention of scientists everywhere: a uranium nucleus could be made to undergo fission—to break into two new atomic nuclei, each roughly half the size of the original—if struck by a neutron. In the process, moreover, a tremendous quantity of energy and several additional neutrons would be released. The implications of this finding were obvious and, with Europe and East Asia in bloody turmoil, of immense importance.

Suppose that both a significant jolt of energy and a pair of neutrons are given off by one fissioning uranium nucleus, and that conditions are such that both of the neutrons instantaneously go on to interact with new uranium nuclei. *Their* fissioning, in turn, will result in the release of four more neutrons (and additional energy), and so on. Once this process gets going, the number of neutrons flying about, and the rate at which energy is being liberated, increases exponentially, as in the progression 1, 2, 4, 8, 16, 32, 64, ... In the explosion of an atomic (fission) bomb, such a chain reaction flashes throughout several kilograms of uranium or plutonium atoms in a slight fraction of a second, and enough energy is released to vaporize a city.

If, on the other hand, neutrons are removed from the uranium at the rate that they are being produced, the resulting controlled reaction can be put to productive use. The energy given off can be harnessed to boil water, and the resulting steam can drive turbines and generate electricity. And among the fission and activation byproducts (the new atoms created when uranium nuclei split apart and emit neutrons) generated in a nuclear reactor are certain radioactive materials that make possible the practice of nuclear medicine imaging.

When a single molecule undergoes a chemical change, such as the loss or gain of a cluster of atoms, a few eV of energy (where the electron volt is the standard measure of energy on the atomic scale) might be given off. The fissioning of one uranium or plutonium nucleus, by contrast, may involve the release of several million eV. Thus, pound for pound, a fission bomb can produce millions of times more energy than its chemical counterpart—and a thermonuclear (fusion) bomb is even worse. That is why the destructive power of a nuclear weapon is expressed in "megatons," or the equivalent of millions of tons, of the conventional explosive TNT.

AIR VENTILATION AND BLOOD PERFUSION STUDIES OF A LUNG EMBOLISM

CASE STUDY

Charlie Steinbeck is a fifty-two-year-old who, for the past twenty years, has driven trucks interstate. During a twelve-hour haul home from Georgia last year, he found his left leg becoming increasingly swollen and uncomfortable. He was jolted awake the next morning by a sharp pain in the lower left side of his chest, stabbing him with each breath, and he began coughing up blood. His wife rushed him to the emergency room where, because his breathing was fast, shallow, and labored, he was immediately given an oxygen mask. A sample of arterial blood soon indicated, indeed, an abnormally low oxygen level.

The ER physician suspected a heart attack, or pneumonia, or a pulmonary embolism (a clot cutting off the flow of blood within part of the lung). During the physical examination, a "rub" could be heard through the stethoscope, like the sound of hands rubbing together, in the lower left portion of the lung, the site of the pain. Mr. Steinbeck's left calf was still swollen and sensitive to the touch. Since his EKG (electrocardiogram) was normal, it was unlikely that he had had a heart attack. A chest X ray taken on a portable machine in the ER appeared normal, indicating that pneumonia was improbable. The signs now pointed to an embolism plugging a major artery of the lung, most likely the result of a blood clot broken off from another one formed recently in the left leg.

A pulmonary embolism would cut off flow of *blood* to a region of the lung (perfusion), but would still allow *air* to enter it (ventilation). Nuclear medicine studies of the flows of blood and air throughout the lungs were therefore performed. A finding that air could reach some region of lung where blood could not go would strongly support the initial diagnosis.

For the lung-ventilation study, Mr. Steinbeck was seated close to the front of a gamma camera, and for a few minutes inhaled radioactive xenon gas. The gas would enter the lungs and fill all parts of it that were not somehow blocked off; a "cold" (abnormally dark) region seen with the gamma camera would indicate an absence of xenon there, and thus a local obstruction to ventilation. This could be caused by a blockage of air passages, the presence of fluids, or the replacement of lung tissue with tumor. But Mr. Steinbeck's ventilation scan was normal (figure 67a). Both lungs appeared clear, with xenon easily washing in and out everywhere.

After the xenon had been expelled, lung perfusion was imaged. The radiopharmacist prepared a solution containing minute clumps of the protein albumin (which occurs normally in blood serum, unclumped), to which were attached radioactive technetium atoms. A small amount of the technetium-labeled macroaggregated albumin (Tc-MAA) was injected into the bloodstream, and the microscopic lumps of it became temporarily lodged in a small but representative fraction of the capillaries of the lung, emitting gamma rays. A cold area in the lower left lung revealed a region that the Tc-MAA (and blood) did not reach (figure 67b).

The pair of isotope tests found a part of the lung that was ventilated but

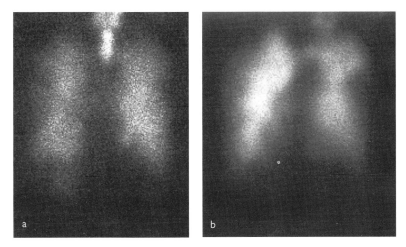

Figure 67. A ventilation/perfusion study. (a) This ventilation scan shows normal distribution of gamma-emitting xenon gas throughout the lung. (b) Dark regions in the lung perfusion study with Tc-MAA, however, reveal that blood (containing the radiopharmaceutical) is not getting to some tissues. Courtesy of Picker International, Inc.

not perfused. Mr. Steinbeck's symptoms, together with his occupation, suggested what had happened: because of the long periods he spent sitting, the flow of blood through the veins of the legs was slowed substantially, increasing the tendency for clots to form there (thrombosis). One piece of clot had broken loose and was swept into the lung, lodging in a narrow pulmonary artery and blocking it off, creating a potentially life-threatening situation.

Mr. Steinbeck was admitted to the hospital, kept on oxygen, and treated intravenously with heparin, a drug that works to prevent the creation of further blood clots. A Doppler ultrasound study (described in chapter 7) was performed on the swollen leg itself, and a finding of decreased blood flow in it provided further support for the diagnosis of pulmonary embolism resulting from thrombosis in a leg vein.

Over time, the clot dissolved, and the renewed perfusion helped some of the lung tissue that was still marginally alive to recover. Mr. Steinbeck was released after a week, but he was maintained on a blood-thinning drug. He still drives a truck, but now wears support stockings and exercises his legs while on the road, and elevates them at the end of the day, all to reduce the likelihood of clot formation. His company has arranged for him to make local deliveries, so that he can avoid long hours of sitting, and he has not had a problem since.

A nuclear medicine picture is made by imaging the gamma rays emitted from a radioactive material that has been introduced into the body and that has concentrated in the organ of interest. Before discussing how the radioactive material gets to the right organ, and how a gamma camera then forms an image, I should explain how the radiation itself comes into being.

An atomic nucleus is made up of protons and neutrons, as discussed in chapter 1 and appendix A. The number of protons, or atomic number, alone determines the element type of the atom—along with virtually all of its mechanical, chemical, optical, electrical, X-ray interaction, and ordinary magnetic characteristics. The behavior of a nucleus, by contrast, depends not only on the particular element, but also on the isotope of that element. The various isotopes of an element have the same number of protons but different numbers of neutrons. The neutron count, in turn, governs whether a particular isotope is radioactive (of interest in nuclear medicine), and also determines its nuclear magnetic properties (of importance in MRI).

It is standard practice to distinguish the several isotopes of an element, when relevant, by appending the total number of protons plus neutrons to the element name or symbol. The nucleus of ordinary, nonradioactive carbon, for example, has six protons and six neutrons, and is written carbon-12, or C-12, or ^{12}C, or even $^{12}_6C$. The radioactive isotope carbon-14, important in the archaeological dating of ancient human artifacts, has six protons and eight neutrons.

There are 2,500 known isotopes of the hundred or so elements, and only 270 of them are inherently stable. The other isotopes are radioactive. Radioactivity is a process whereby an excited, unstable nucleus drops to a state of lower energy and (often) of greater stability. There are a number of ways this can happen, but for conventional nuclear medicine, only one is important: in *gamma emission*, a nucleus de-excites through the release of a high-energy gamma-ray photon. Recall that gamma rays differ from X rays only in their origin—whereas the X rays used in imaging are produced in the collisions of high-velocity electrons with the anode of an X-ray tube, gamma rays come from spontaneous nuclear transformations.

Although amounts of most substances are measured in units of weight or volume, radioactive materials are quantified in terms of "activity." The activity of a sample of radioactive material is defined as the number of decay events taking place in it per unit of time. (The activity of a sample is not the same thing as the number of radioactive nuclei present, but it is

The other common forms of radioactivity are the emission of a beta particle (an electron), a positron (a positively charged electron), or an alpha particle (a tightly bound complex of two protons and two neutrons, i.e., the nucleus of a normal helium atom) from an unstable nucleus. Alpha and beta emissions find no use in medical imaging, but if they occur within the body, they will deposit radiation dose. Positrons play a limited, but interesting, role in PET, as will be discussed later in this chapter.

proportional to that number.) The international metric unit of activity is the becquerel (Bq), defined as one nuclear decay event per second. More familiar in the United States is the curie (Ci), where one curie means thirty-seven billion decays per second (1 Ci = 3.7×10^{10} Bq). In most nuclear medicine studies, with some important exceptions, a few millicuries of radioactive material are administered to the patient. (A millicurie is one thousandth of a curie, abbreviated "mCi.")

The activity of a sample of a radioisotope will fall to half its initial value over a period of time, called the *half-life*, that is characteristic of that isotope. The half-life of carbon-14 is 5,730 years, for example, whereas that of technetium-99m, the workhorse of any nuclear medicine department, is six hours. If a patient receives a 4 mCi injection of Tc-99m at 6 A.M., then 2 mCi will remain in the body at noon, 1 mCi at 6 P.M., 0.5 mCi at midnight, and so on, assuming that none is lost in urine, perspiration, etc. The activity of a radioisotope sample is said to decay exponentially over time, as you would see in figure 22 if you relabeled the vertical axis as "Relative Activity" and the horizontal axis as "Time (hours)," with its scale marks labeled 0, 6, 12, 18, 24, 30.

Nothing is decaying in the ordinary sense of the word. "Decay" refers here to the nuclear transformations of radionuclei (changing them into different nuclei) that take place over time—hence to a decline in their number.

WHERE IN THE BODY DOES THE RADIOPHARMACEUTICAL GO?

Nuclear medicine makes use of radiopharmaceuticals, special radioactive materials that display two key features: an injected or inhaled sample of such a material is taken up preferentially by a specific organ; and from there, it emits gamma rays that can be detected and imaged from outside the body (see figure 12). Any irregularity in the spatial distribution of radioactive material within the organ, as revealed by a gamma camera, may indicate a pathologic condition.

A typical radiopharmaceutical is a solution containing special molecules or microscopic particles made up of two components, a chemical agent and a radioactive atom. The agent is designed to concentrate in a particular organ, and perhaps even at different rates in healthy and abnormal tissues of the organ. This uptake can occur in different ways. Examination of the blood vessel system of the lungs is made possible through a temporary blockage of about 1 percent of the lung capillaries by microscopic clumps of macroaggregated albumin (MAA); the albumin particles break down soon thereafter, and are quickly flushed out of the lung. In studies of the thyroid, small molecules containing radioactive iodine are actively transported into cells of the gland by biochemical pumps in the cell walls. Tiny particles of radio-labeled sulfur allow study of the liver and spleen and bone marrow because scavenger cells there trap and engulf them. And lately there has been particular interest in certain monoclonal antibodies as agents, mass-produced proteins designed to bind to specific diseased cells.

The second constituent of a radiopharmaceutical is a radioactive atom that is part of, or can be made to attach to, the agent. It can thereby go along for the ride to the target organ and, from there, emit gamma-ray photons of a suitable energy. Although several dozen radioisotopes are used routinely in the nuclear medicine department, the most common one, by far, is technetium-99m. Tc-99m has physical characteristics that make it nearly ideal for imaging. It emits only gamma rays, no useless (but ionizing) alphas or betas. The energy of its gamma-ray photons (140,000 eV) is such that they will likely escape the body but then be stopped and detected by the gamma camera. Tc-99m can be delivered every day to the clinic by a commercial vendor, or it can be obtained by flushing sterile salt water through a technetium generator ("cow") supplied weekly by the vendor. Its six-hour half-life provides sufficient time for preparation of radiopharmaceuticals in the clinic, and it can easily and rapidly be attached to a variety of agents that come in kits. You simply add radioisotope solution from the cow to the material from the kit, heat and stir, and mumble the requisite incantation; you then load the right quantity of it into a syringe, double-check it with an activity-measuring instrument, inject it into the patient, and take the image a little later. But the half-life is also short enough for the gamma irradiation of the patient (and of those nearby) to diminish rapidly after the study is completed.

A nuclear medicine image is of relatively low spatial resolution and reveals only the rough shape and size of the organ under consideration. But if a portion of the organ fails to take up the radiopharmaceutical, or is missing, or is obscured by overlying abnormal tissues, the corresponding region of the image appears dark. Likewise, any part of the organ that absorbs more radiopharmaceutical than normal will glow especially brightly on the display. Thus a nuclear medicine image provides information on the physiologic status and pathologies of an organ, rather than on its anatomic details.

THE NUTS AND BOLTS OF A GAMMA CAMERA

Nuclear medicine involves the sensing of trace amounts of radioactive material that tend to end up in specific organs. A simple device that can accomplish this task is the scintillation detector, a crystal of fluorescent material (such as sodium iodide, NaI) optically coupled to a photomultiplier tube. When excited by a gamma-ray photon, the crystal produces a burst of light. The photomultiplier generates a jolt of electricity whenever it registers such a scintillation—and the brighter the flash, the greater the voltage kick of the pulse.

Technetium, with atomic number 43, is one of the three elements lighter than uranium that do not occur naturally in significant amounts on Earth (the others are promethium and astatine), and the first to have been created artificially, in 1937. The *m* in Tc-99m stands for "metastable," which means, for our purposes, that it emits only gamma rays, no betas or alphas.

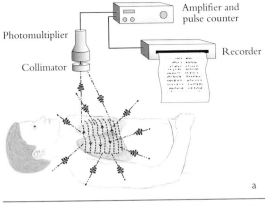

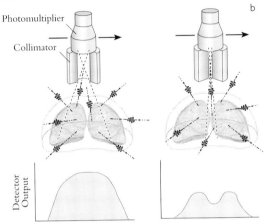

Figure 68. Rectilinear scanner. (a) A collimator and gamma-ray detector are moved together in a raster pattern over the patient, and the pen of the printer mimics that motion. Every time a gamma ray makes it through the hole in the collimator and is detected, the pen leaves a dot of ink on the paper. (b) A fundamental trade-off: a smaller-bore collimator, which yields better resolution, also has lower sensitivity, requiring either the intake of more radiopharmaceutical by the patient or slower scanning (hence more time).

Before the advent of the gamma camera, maps of radioisotope uptake were produced with the rectilinear scanner (figure 68a). A scanner consisted of a scintillation detector with a collimator (a thick block of lead, through which one or several narrow, straight channels are drilled) on its front end. Only those few gamma rays that happened to be heading exactly along a channel reached the detector. The collimator / detector assembly was swept in a raster pattern, back and forth across while moving slowly down the patient. A pen held over a sheet of paper was linked to the collimator / detector and made to trace out the same path; every time a gamma ray registered, the pen tapped the paper. The density of ink dots anywhere on the paper indicated the rate at which gamma rays were emerging from the corresponding part of the body, and hence, the concentration of radiopharmaceutical below the surface there.

Introduced in the late 1950s, the gamma camera is much more flexible and efficient than the rectilinear scanner (figure 69a). A gamma camera detects and records gamma rays much as an ordinary camera records visible light. But since gamma rays cannot be focused, the role of the lens

Figure 68b suggests a fundamental and important trade-off in nuclear medicine image quality: a larger-diameter collimator channel will let more gamma rays through but will allow less accurate location of their source. Thus an improvement in detector sensitivity is paid for in loss of spatial resolution. There are many such trade-offs in every imaging modality, and an important job of equipment developers, and of medical staffs, is to strike the best possible balances among them.

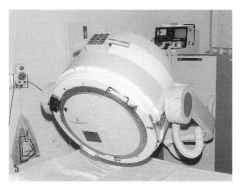
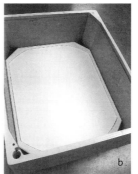
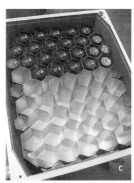

Figure 69. A conventional gamma camera. (a) The flat plate with the handles, on the front of the camera, is the collimator. (b) The large, thin sodium iodide (NaI) scintillation crystal (c) is observed by an array of up to a hundred photomultipliers. (d) The site of an individual scintillation is determined by the array of photomultiplier tubes: the closer any tube is to a scintillation, the brighter it appears and the higher the voltage of the pulse it produces. By weighting the pulse voltages from all the tubes, the camera's scintillation-location logic circuit can ascertain where in the crystal the flash occurred. Figures b and c courtesy of Picker International, Inc.

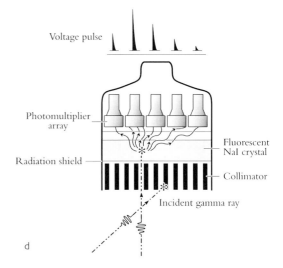

Voltage pulse

Photomultiplier array

Radiation shield

Fluorescent NaI crystal

Collimator

Incident gamma ray

d

is played by a multihole collimator, consisting of hundreds of small-diameter channels, separated from one another by thin walls of lead foil. A gamma ray that does not travel along the straight and narrow is absorbed in the lead, as with a radiographic grid. Behind the collimator is a large (up to twenty-four inches in diameter), thin, single crystal of sodium iodide doped with trace amounts of other materials to enhance its fluorescence characteristics (figure 69b). A gamma ray that does manage to pass along a channel of the collimator and interact with the crystal produces a burst of light. The crystal, in turn, is observed by a honeycomb array of up to 100 separate photomultiplier tubes, each of which will sense any nearby scintillation event (figure 69c). Together, they can determine where within the crystal the gamma ray struck, hence where in the body it came from. This information is processed by a computer, and the composite image is displayed on a monitor.

You are probably wondering how the gamma camera ascertains where the gamma ray landed. A scintillation in the sodium iodide crystal elicits a voltage pulse from each of the neighboring photomultiplier tubes (figure

69d). The nearer a tube is to the site of the flash, the greater its apparent brightness, and the larger the voltage pulse from the tube. The scintillation-location logic circuit knows the position of every photomultiplier tube and, by intercomparing the voltage pulses from all of them, it can estimate where in the sodium iodide crystal the burst of light actually occurred, to better than a centimeter.

Accumulating data through hundreds of collimator holes, rather than the one or few of a scanner, reduces both the imaging time and the amount of radiopharmaceutical that has to be given to the patient. And the ability of a gamma camera (obviously missing in a scanner) to observe an entire anatomic region of interest continuously makes feasible the study of time-dependent phenomena, such as the beating of a heart.

NUCLEAR CARDIOLOGY: FREEZING THE HEART'S MOTIONS

Nuclear medicine offers noninvasive, safe alternatives to some cardiac catheterization studies. It also provides nontraumatic ways of following the response of the heart to surgery or other kinds of therapy, both in the resting state and under mild physical stress.

Physiologically, the element thallium acts much like potassium, which tends to concentrate within muscle cells. The uptake of thallium by a muscle is roughly proportional to the rate of blood flow to it, and in addition it depends on the muscle's state of health. The amount of thallium uptake by myocardial (heart muscle) cells, in particular, can be significantly decreased by ischemia (reduced blood flow) resulting from coronary artery disease or from myocardial infarction (a heart attack, in which some heart muscle is deprived of oxygen, and its cells begin to die). So a nuclear medicine study of the heart typically involves a search for areas of reduced thallium uptake by cardiac muscle.

A normal gamma camera image of the heart would be hopelessly blurred by its motion, so techniques have been devised to "freeze" that movement. A multiple-gated acquisition (MUGA) cardiac study takes advantage of the regular, repetitive nature of the heart's pumping action, and works somewhat like a stroboscope. It stores separate images that correspond to different segments of the heartbeat cycle in a set of two dozen or so separate frames, three of which are shown in figure 70. Each frame is partitioned into a matrix, typically of $128 \times 128 = 16,000$ or so pixels. The first frame, triggered "on" by the voltage spike that occurs once every heartbeat in the patient's electrocardiogram (EKG) signal, accumulates counts for, say, forty milliseconds. Any gamma ray event in the first $40/1000$ of a second simply increases the level of brightness at the appropriate pixel, as with any ordinary nuclear medicine image. After that,

The gamma camera can also add up the pulses from all the detectors to estimate the total amount of light produced in a scintillation event. But the intensity of a burst of light is proportional to the energy of the gamma ray responsible for it, and gamma ray energies are radioisotope-specific. This energy-specificity allows the gamma camera to accept only scintillations from the imaging isotope, rejecting visible-light noise from other sources.

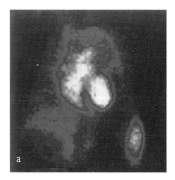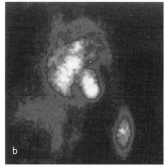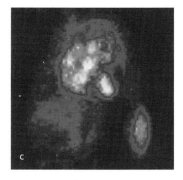

Figure 70. A multi-gated (MUGA) cardiac study, with the timing provided by an electrocardiogram. The cardiac cycle is partitioned into two dozen or so brief periods, with one image frame corresponding to each. A frame collects data for only about forty milliseconds at a time, but does so for many consecutive beats of the heart. Three frames are shown here. Courtesy of Picker International, Inc.

the second frame takes over, for the same length of time, then the third, and so on. This stepping procedure continues for the two dozen frames, long enough to cover one heartbeat. Then the next EKG spike starts the whole business over again, back at frame 1. Although little data is obtained during a single cycle, several hundred repetitions result in cumulative frame images with adequate numbers of gamma ray counts.

After all the frames have stored sufficient information, any one of them can provide an unblurred image. A dark area may indicate a region of diminished blood flow or damaged heart muscle; likewise, abnormal patterns of blood flow observed during exercise may suggest coronary artery disease. Alternatively, one can view a rather dazzling motion picture of the heart as it pulses by repeatedly displaying all the frames in rapid sequence.

Reconstruction computations are similar to, but more complex than, those of CT. The detected signal depends not only on the distribution of gamma-emitting material within the organ of interest (usually of primary clinical importance in nuclear medicine), but also on the absorption of photons by the other tissues (as with CT—but for SPECT, this does not help create the image, it just muddies the waters).

SINGLE PHOTON EMISSION COMPUTED TOMOGRAPHY

Single photon emission computed tomography (SPECT), a cross between standard nuclear medicine and X-ray computed tomography, creates CT-like, nuclear medicine slice-images. These can be examined individually, or stacked to create a three-dimensional picture (figure 71a). Several standard gamma camera heads, mounted on a single supporting gantry (figure 71b), are rotated slowly around the patient, and data are acquired at a number of angles.

Many new commercial gamma imagers are capable of performing SPECT, and clinical researchers are exploring its potential medical benefits. The obvious advantage is that SPECT allows the physician to visualize an organ in three quite different ways—as a set of individual tomographic slices (as with CT); as a solid object in three dimensions

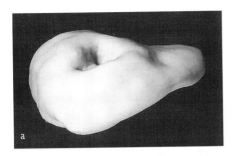

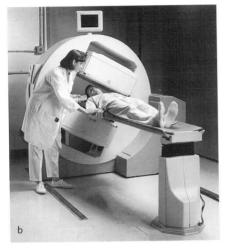

Figure 71. SPECT uses gamma camera information collected from a number of different viewing angles to produce CT-like slices. (a) These can be stacked to create a three-dimensional image, as with this liver study that reveals an indentation caused by an abnormal growth. (b) Each of the two heads of this SPECT imager can alone serve as a standard gamma camera. Courtesy of Picker International, Inc.

viewed, perhaps, as it rotates; or as a standard two-dimensional nuclear medicine image (but as seen from any angle). This capability alone may be more than enough to justify a SPECT machine's somewhat greater acquisition cost.

POSITRON EMISSION TOMOGRAPHY

Positron emission tomography (PET) is a subfield of nuclear medicine that has long been of considerable research value. PET was initially employed primarily for imaging variations in the flow of blood and in the rate of glucose metabolism throughout the normal and abnormal brain, and in studies of cerebral activity. More recently, it has been finding important clinical applications as well.

As with conventional nuclear medicine or SPECT, PET involves the detection of high-energy photons. But PET differs notably in three regards: the photons are not emitted directly by the nucleus; they happen to be of much higher energy (a half million eV) than is normally employed in nuclear medicine; and they are always detected in pairs.

PET scanning exploits the predisposition of a few radioisotopes to emit positrons, particles that are completely identical to electrons in all re-

There are no positrons zipping around within the nucleus anxious to escape, any more than there is an omelet waiting to happen inside an egg. A nuclear transformation takes place, in effect, in which a proton briefly metamorphoses into a neutron and a positron (and a neutrino, which plays no role in medicine); the positron (and neutrino) are on their way before the process has time to reverse itself, leaving behind a nucleus with one fewer proton and one more neutron.

Positron annihilation provides a lovely example of Einstein's formula, $E = mc^2$, for keeping track of quantities of mass, m, and energy, E, when one form is being transformed into the other. The equation indicates that an annihilating positron and electron will create a pair of photons of 511,000 eV energy each, as is confirmed by measurement. The constant c represents the speed of light.

An attractive feature of F-18 for medical purposes is its half-life of nearly two hours—much longer than those of C-11 (20 min.), N-13 (10 min.), or O-15 (2 min.)—which allows time for its chemical incorporation into complex metabolites for imaging.

gards except for their positive charge. After it is ejected from a nucleus, the typical positron slows down over a millimeter or so in tissue and then bumps into an ordinary electron. The positron and electron are *antiparticles:* when they meet, they instantaneously annihilate one another, creating a pair of "annihilation" photons with about the same energy but traveling in opposite directions. The two new photons will sometimes be detected at exactly the same time by two separate detectors on opposite sides of the patient—indicating that the positron-emitter was located somewhere along the straight line joining them (figure 72). Simultaneous detection of a sufficient number of such pairs of annihilation photons, from multiple angles, yields enough information to create a two- or three-dimensional PET map of the uptake of the radioisotope with a resolution of about one half centimeter.

A big reason for the interest in PET is that the list of positron-emitting nuclei happens to include isotopes of carbon, nitrogen, and oxygen, all elements that are major constituents of tissues. These have been prepared for PET studies as gaseous oxygen, water, carbon monoxide, carbon dioxide, and ammonia, and some have been incorporated into more complex molecules such as sugars and amino acids. These can then be used to trace various biochemical pathways. Water (H_2O) and molecular oxygen (O_2) , each containing one atom of unstable oxygen-15, for example, have been used extensively to monitor blood flow and oxygen metabolism in the brain—processes, it has been found, that can be influenced by diseases and by some physical and mental stimuli, as shown in figure 13b.

One particular combination of positron-emitting radionuclide plus agent is stirring up its own nuclear medicine revolution. Although not much ordinary, nonradioactive fluorine occurs naturally in the body, the unstable isotope fluorine-18 can be readily substituted for hydrogen (or hydroxyl, -OH) in a number of biomolecules, such as the sugar glucose. PET can then observe as cells metabolize F-18 fluorodeoxyglucose (FDG), much as they would normal glucose. FDG is effective in detecting and imaging certain cancers of the brain, head, neck, breast, lung, liver, and colon. It is also finding an important application in monitoring the course of cancer therapy. CT or MRI can reveal whether the size of a malignancy is changing (one way or the other) following the beginning of treatment, but the effects of radiation or drugs may be apparent much earlier from alterations in the tumor's metabolism. These can be detected by PET, allowing the treatment to be adjusted sooner—and a small time difference can be critical.

In a quite different role, PET with FDG may sometimes be better than standard nuclear cardiology in predicting the outcome of cardiac bypass surgery. PET reflects the basic metabolic activity (in particular, the rate of

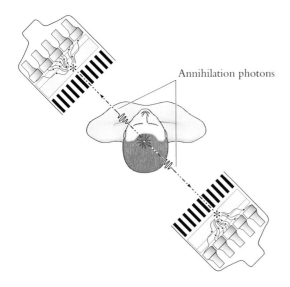

Annihilation photons

Figure 72. Immediately after being emitted from the radiopharmaceutical, a positron collides with an electron. They annihilate one another, and the two high-energy photons resulting from this event speed off in opposite directions. The simultaneous triggering of two separate detectors of a PET camera then can reveal the line of flight of the two photons—and the original positron-emitting nucleus must have been somewhere along that line. The region of intersection of many such lines, for many camera angles, delineates the original distribution of the radiopharmaceutical.

glucose consumption) of cardiac muscle after a heart attack. Tissues that are too damaged to take up thallium, and that earlier might have been considered beyond hope, may now be seen with PET to be functional enough to recover, following the return of a good supply of oxygen; so PET offers a second chance to some patients who, before, would not have been considered candidates for surgery.

Several technological developments, too, are helping to draw PET out of the laboratory and into the clinical mainstream. It has long been an exciting and productive research tool, but it is expensive. A standard PET scanner is elaborate, with a sticker price two to four times that of a CT machine, and yet it has rather narrow diagnostic utility. Also, because of their short half-lives, most of the positron-emitting radionuclides have had to be produced on-site, generally by means of a complex and pricey cyclotron. But PET costs are dropping rapidly now, for two reasons. First, manufacturers of SPECT imagers have come to realize that a somewhat thicker sodium iodide crystal not only will still work well enough for technetium, but also can perform adequately with the higher-energy photons coming from positron annihilation. So they are now building two-headed SPECT machines that employ scintillation crystals thick enough to carry out PET as well. A combined SPECT / PET device may not be of absolutely optimal design for either application alone, but being able to do both kinds of study reasonably well on one relatively inexpensive machine has great appeal. Second, fluorine-18 is becoming readily available from local suppliers in many cities—you no longer have to make your own positron emitter with an expensive cyclotron.

The number of medical centers with PET capability is still small, and it remains to be seen how cost-effective positron imaging will become. But with the advent of relatively affordable SPECT / PET cameras and the greater accessibility of radiopharmaceuticals, I would venture a guess that the field will continue to grow briskly.

NUCLEAR CARDIOLOGY FOR A MILD HEART ATTACK

Kilauea Liliuokalani is an outwardly relaxed, but highly energetic and intensely focused professor of anthropology at the University of Maui. Forty-two years old, he neither drinks excessively nor smokes, exercises regularly, and has always enjoyed excellent health. But both his father and his grandfather died suddenly at early ages, presumably because of heart disease, and for many years he has been mildly apprehensive about possible cardiac problems.

Dr. Liliuokalani recently experienced a new, vague chest discomfort—a certain tightness—while playing a vigorous game of tennis. There was no pain in his arm or jaw, and the sensation in his chest vanished soon after the match. Even though he thought it was probably only indigestion, he paid his internist a visit.

EKG and blood tests showed no evidence of a heart attack. But the internist was not entirely comfortable with these results, and she referred her patient to a cardiologist. The cardiologist agreed with the internist's suspicions that the symptoms might be attributable to coronary artery disease. This could lead, with physical exertion, to a reduction in the flow of oxygen through the coronary arteries to the heart muscle itself, giving rise to discomfort but not yet killing any heart muscle cells. To confirm this diagnosis, Dr. Liliuokalani underwent a stress electrocardiogram, in which the EKG tracing is monitored both before and while the patient runs on a treadmill. There was a slight, possible difference between the two EKGs, but the outcome of this test was equivocal for diminished blood flow to the heart muscle.

One possible next step could be cardiac catheterization. But the cardiologist felt that valuable further information could be obtained noninvasively (and hence more safely) and less expensively through a nuclear medicine cardiac stress study. If that clearly proved negative, then the catheterization would not be necessary unless the problem worsened.

Soon after checking into the nuclear medicine department, Dr. Liliuokalani was pedaling away on a stationary exercise bicycle close to the face of a gamma camera. After he was given an injection of radioactive thallium, multi-gated studies were carried out both immediately and long after light exercise. The differential uptake of thallium can be seen in a pair of views of the heart just after exercise (figure 73a), and two hours after

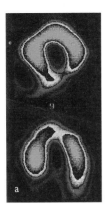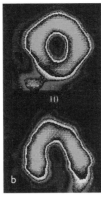

Figure 73. Coronary artery disease. (a) This stress test shows two views of a region of heart muscle that takes up too little thallium isotope during exercise. (b) Following two hours of rest, the heart appears "normal" again. This difference is suggestive of a partial blockage of the coronary artery that supplies the region. Courtesy of Kevin Nealon, Chevy Chase, Md.

(figure 73b). The changes in the patterns indicate an abnormally low flow of blood to part of the heart wall, probably attributable to a partial blockage of one of the coronary arteries.

Soon thereafter, Dr. Liliuokalani underwent cardiac catheterization. In the cardiac cath lab, a catheter was threaded from the main artery of the leg, up the aorta, and into the left coronary artery under fluoroscopy. A blockage in the left anterior descending (LAD) coronary artery, similar to what was seen in figure 34, was easily located with contrast agent. An intense beam of laser light emerging from the tip of a fiber-optic cable attached to the catheter produced heat that eliminated much of the built-up plaque, and there were no complications.

Within days, Dr. Liliuokalani was a greatly relieved anthropologist. A carefully selected diet, anticholesterol medication, and continued exercise will help keep him feeling that way.

7

Shadows from Echoes

ULTRASOUND

People have used echoes of high-frequency sound to find or track invisible objects, such as submarines, for nearly a hundred years. Other members of the animal kingdom, some that must hunt and find their way around in dark and murky worlds, have been doing so for aeons.

OF BATS AND BOATS: GETTING AROUND IN THE DARK

Among the most successful of echo-locating creatures have been some species of dolphins and killer whales. Many of the underwater sounds with which they communicate are familiar—the low-pitched barks, clicks, whistles, and songs that lie within the range of human hearing. But they also produce brief pulses of ultrasound, up to 200,000 cycles per second in frequency, which they project from the forehead and lower jaw in a narrowly defined beam. Their perception of the resulting echoes, apparently mediated through the jaw and throat rather than the ears, is highly directional. The echo-locational skills of a bottle-nosed dolphin are impressive: it can detect a golf ball several hundred feet away, discriminate among balls of slightly different sizes, sense the presence of fine wire, and even tell a copper disk from an aluminum one, all by sound echoes alone.

Bats, unlike dolphins, aren't exactly everyone's idea of sweet and cuddly, but they do have some redeeming qualities. They produce prodigious amounts of guano, an important source of fertilizer in some societies; they

The acoustic advantage, it should be noted, is not entirely with the bats. To ward off predators, some moths have managed to acquire a singularly foul taste, and they advertise their undesirability with distinctive coloration and markings. Such a strictly visual approach, of course, cannot work against nocturnal hunters such as insect-eating bats. So a few species of moths have evolved a remarkable additional layer of defense —the ability not only to sense a bat's pulses, but also to reply with distinctive clicks that warn, "I'm no bat snack! Take a bite out of me, and you'll be sorry!" And in one of Mother Nature's more cunning moves, even several *nice*-tasting (depending on your gastronomic predilections) moths have learned to mimic the clicks of their inedible cousins.

consume insects voraciously; and their ability to navigate by sound borders on the unbelievable. For several centuries, it has been known that a flying bat can avoid obstacles if deprived of sight, but not if its ears are plugged; it was not until 1939, however, that actual bat cries were detected and recorded. These come as short pulses, we have since learned, up to a hundred per second, that extend in frequency from 12,000 Hz (near the top of the audible range for humans) up to ten or more times higher. A vibrating membrane in the larynx produces the sound and, in some species, a parabolically shaped mouth focuses it into a narrow beam, as with the curved mirror of a flashlight. A bat's vocalizations can be quite complex in design, with significant variation in intensity and frequency during a pulse; this may be because a signal that includes a wide band of frequencies will generate echoes rich in information content, since sounds of different frequencies are reflected and absorbed in different amounts by different objects and materials.

A bat's data-processing system is even more awe-inspiring. While constantly comparing the slightly different signals that reach its two ears separately, a bat must distinguish the relevant sounds from all background noises, including extraneous echoes that it and its fellow travelers have produced. It has but a few thousandths of a second to analyze and interpret the incoming data while it and perhaps its target are bobbing and weaving at high speeds in three dimensions. Yet with sound alone, a bat can locate and catch something as small and quick as a fruit fly.

Perhaps inspired by the remarkable capabilities of other species, humans began working on acoustic echo-location before World War I, ini-

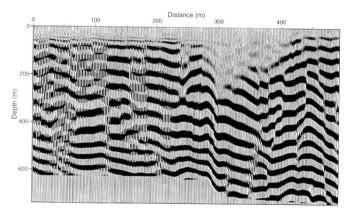

Figure 74. This seismic reflection section of some land in Arizona shows boundaries between basalt, through which sound passes rapidly, and limestone, sandstone, and other lower-velocity rocks. Borehole samples can provide such information at one location, but seismic studies reveal faults, fractures, caverns, and other features in three dimensions. Courtesy of Michael Rymer, U.S. Geological Survey.

tially to watch for icebergs and then to hunt submarines. Active sonar (an acronym of sound navigation and ranging) has evolved considerably since then, in large part because of the fast-pulse electronics technology developed during and since World War II for radar (radio detection and ranging). As with bats and dolphins, the basic idea in sonar is to produce short, high-frequency pulses and detect their echoes. The orientation of the ultrasound beam at the time of pulse transmission gives the bearing of a target object; the measured return time of the echo, together with the known velocity of sound in water, yields its distance; and the acoustic signature of the echo pulses may provide information on the size, movement, and other characteristics of the target.

Sonar has had nonmilitary applications as well, such as in charting the seafloor and navigating by way of such charts. Likewise, modern fish-finding systems use sonar, as do instruments for oil and gas exploration and studies of geologic formations (figure 74). But the spin-off from sonar technology best known to the public is ultrasound medical imaging.

ULTRASOUND OF AN INFLAMED GALL BLADDER

CASE STUDY

Sylvia Sexton is a forty-three-year-old corporate lawyer and single mother of three teenage children. She has a history of emotional difficulties (mild chronic anxiety and depression) for which she will not accept treatment. She is five feet four inches tall and pushing 180 pounds; aside from being considerably overweight, she has always enjoyed good physical health.

For the past half year, however, Ms. Sexton has been experiencing an uneasy, bloated feeling in her right upper abdomen, especially after eating fatty foods. Over the last month, this sensation, and a new stabbing pain in the same area, have increased significantly in severity, and Ms. Sexton began to worry that she might be having mild heart attacks. To her internist, her symptoms suggested the presence of gall stones. The gall bladder is a small sac that stores bile, a fluid produced by the liver to help in the digestion of fats, and releases it into the intestines as needed. Occasionally some of the bile congeals into small hard rocks that can cause considerable pain when they attempt to exit the gall bladder through its narrow neck.

The easiest, quickest, and cheapest way to confirm such a diagnosis is by way of an ultrasound. After fasting since midnight, Ms. Sexton showed up early at the radiology department of her local hospital. As she lay on her back on the examination table, an ultrasound technologist rubbed a slippery gel on her abdomen. A thin veneer of it provided good acoustic contact between the ultrasound transducer and her body and allowed the de-

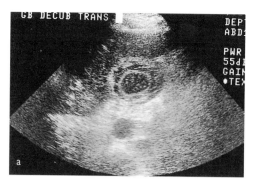 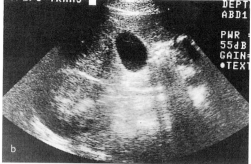

Figure 75. B-mode ultrasound of a gall bladder revealing (a) no gall stones—rather, an abnormally thick wall and the suggestion that the organ contains a thick sludge. (b) After treatment, the gall bladder appears normal.

vice to glide around smoothly. The transducer, which somewhat resembles a microphone, actually functions part of the time as one. Driven by the ultrasound transmitter, it produces bursts of very high frequency sound waves (which the patient neither hears nor feels) that enter the body and reflect off tissue interfaces within; the transducer then detects the resulting echoes and, from their timing and strengths, the system's receiver and computer create a digital image (see figure 15).

As the ultrasound technologist moved the transducer about, he identified shapes on a nearby TV screen that, with a bit of imagination, Ms. Sexton could visualize as separate organs, including the liver and gall bladder. He stored what he considered to be the most diagnostically informative images, and had the laser printer produce some of them on radiographic film. The whole procedure took about an hour and caused no discomfort.

Several hours later, the hospital's radiologist most experienced with ultrasound read the films and sent a report to Ms. Sexton's physician. Instead of revealing solid objects or normal fluid (which would produce no echoes at all), the ultrasound images showed that the gall bladder was filled with some sort of sludgy material (figure 75a). Also, its wall appeared abnormally thick, indicating significant chronic inflammation, presumably arising from irritation caused by the sludge.

The current standard approach to this problem, laparoscopic cholecystectomy, involves making a few very small incisions in the patient's abdomen and snipping out the offending organ—a fast and safe procedure. Ms. Sexton was extremely anxious about anesthesia and surgery, however, and insisted that the problem be treated medically instead. Within several months, medication and proper diet had caused the abnormal contents of the gall bladder to dissolve, and the resulting decrease in irritation led to a reduction and eventual vanishing of the inflammation. A

A laparoscope is an endoscope designed specifically for seeing within the abdominal cavity through a small surgical slit; *-ectomy* means removal, and *cholecyst-* refers to the gall bladder.

repeat study proved normal (figure 75b). Ms. Sexton is keeping to her diet, in particular restricting her intake of fats, and it is unlikely that the problem will recur.

MEDICAL ULTRASOUND IS MUCH LIKE SONAR

With all the other technologies described in this book, the radiation that interacts with body tissues is electromagnetic energy. With ultrasound, it consists of something quite different: high-frequency sound waves.

Sound consists of periodic mechanical disturbances, waves of compression and decompression, that propagate through a medium such as air or water. The middle C bar of a xylophone, for example, vibrates 261.6 times each second, and it creates local disturbances of the air around it primarily of this frequency. As the wood or metal plate resonates, it alternately increases and reduces the pressure in the air immediately adjacent, which pushes and pulls on the next layer of air, in effect, and so on (figure 76). The disturbance radiates outward, and eventually causes displacements of your eardrum, resulting in the sensation of a sound.

Medical ultrasound works much like sonar, sending out high-frequency sound and gaining information from the resulting echoes. The essential tasks are to produce precisely sculpted, high-frequency electrical pulses; transform them into localized bundles of high-frequency sound energy that radiate out from the transducer in a preordained direction; pick up the much fainter echoes; turn these back into electrical signals; and process and analyze the signals and extract the relevant information content.

Also present are small-amplitude harmonics —vibrations occurring at integer multiples (i.e., two times, three times, etc.) of the base frequency. The middle C of a piano is distinguishable from that of a violin because of differences in their harmonic makeup.

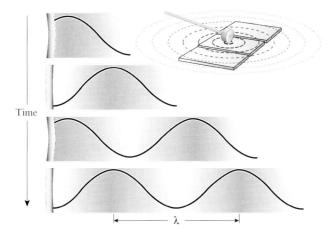

Figure 76. Waves of increased and decreased air pressure are produced by a vibrating plate, membrane, or string. These propagate through the air and drive the eardrum, thereby triggering some motion-sensitive nerve cells. These convey an indication of the event to the brain, resulting in the sensation of sound.

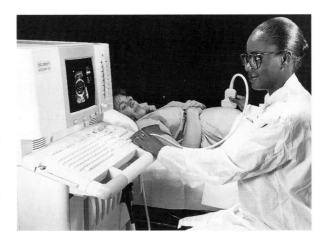

Figure 77. A modern ultrasound system (see figure 15). High-frequency electrical pulses generated by the transmitter are converted into mechanical vibrations by the piezoelectric elements of a transducer, held by the technologist. The transducer, acting as a microphone, then picks up any echoes originating within the body and converts them into electrical signals, which are processed by the receiver and computer for display. Courtesy of Acuson, Inc.

At the heart of a typical transducer are many small, thin, flat wafers of piezoelectric material that generate and detect the mechanical vibrations. A piezoelectric substance is one that deforms slightly when subjected to an electric field and, conversely, produces an electric voltage when it is compressed or bent.

In clinical ultrasound, as seen in figure 77, a transmitter produces a short pulse (typically a few millionths of a second) of high-frequency electrical oscillations (one to ten MHz, or million cycles per second). The transducer, acting like a loudspeaker, converts this electric signal into a pulse of mechanical vibrations of about the same frequency and duration. With the transducer pressed firmly against the patient's body, and acoustically coupled to it with gel or oil, the pulse of ultrasound energy enters with little reflection at the skin, and propagates inward through soft tissues and fluids. Then, quiescent and acting as a microphone, the same (or another) transducer senses any reflected, much weaker pulses of ultrasound, and transforms them back into electrical signals. Echoes from distinct organs, blood vessels, and other structures are amplified and processed by the receiver, and are sent to a computer, which keeps track of their return times and amplitudes.

About a thousandth of a second later, another pulse is produced and sent off in a slightly different direction through the body, and the whole process begins anew. From echo data generated in this fashion, the computer can create a CT-like image in "real time"—you can actually watch the arms and legs of a fetus move about, or see a heart valve open and close.

Ultrasound is useful in the study of soft tissues and organs that are radiologically too similar (i.e., whose X-ray attenuation coefficient values are too much alike) to provide adequate X-ray image contrast. Also, Doppler ultrasound can detect and monitor the flow (or lack thereof) of blood in the arteries and veins, as will be seen below. Ultrasound is employed extensively for obstetric / gynecologic, cardiac, vascular, and general abdominal imaging. If a diagnostic question can be resolved by any of several modalities, then ultrasound may be the one of choice because of its low cost and the absence of ionizing radiation.

WHAT DETERMINES HOW STRONG AN ECHO WILL BE?

When traversing a homogeneous material, such as the fluid within a cyst or large blood vessel, an ultrasound pulse simply dissipates its energy as heat as it penetrates to greater depths, and no echoes are produced. The cyst or vessel appears uniformly blank, with no internal structure. But if the beam passes through several different organs or dissimilar tissues, energy is reflected at interfaces between them. The time of return of an echo back to the surface is proportional to the depth within the body of the interface that produced it. The echo's intensity depends not only on that, but also on the degree of difference in physical properties of the materials on the two sides of the interface.

Sharp echoes will be produced at a sizable and relatively flat boundary between any two materials that have significantly different physical characteristics. The amount of reflection that occurs at such an interface depends largely on the differences in the elasticities (or the compressibilities, which are closely related) and densities of the media on the two sides of it. These are the two determinants of the speed of sound in a fluid, as well, so we can also think of reflection (and refraction) as occurring where the velocity of the waves changes abruptly. The larger the disconnect in elasticity or density, or sound velocity, the greater the fraction of incident ultrasound that is reflected. If, on the other hand, the two materials have similar acoustic properties, most of the ultrasound energy will pass from one to the other, and any echoes produced there will be weak.

An analogy may be helpful here. If you were to give one end of a long wire coil or rope a hefty shake, a ripple would run along it (figure 78). If the far end of the coil is attached to a heavier or more rigid grade of coil, a smaller ripple will reflect at the juncture and head back toward you, while another wave, also smaller than the original, will continue on along the second coil. Likewise, there will be a partial reflection if the far end is attached to a lighter-weight coil, or a more springy one. But if the coil happens to interface smoothly with another coil of exactly the same type, the ripple just keeps on going. The same thing happens when ultrasound energy comes to a boundary surface between two materials, as opposed to when it continues on through a homogeneous medium.

The amounts of energy reflection occurring at several important kinds of tissue interfaces are shown in table 1. As would be expected from the large differences in density and compressibility, ultrasound energy does not pass readily across tissue-air or tissue-bone boundaries. Ultrasound is therefore of little use in examining lung or adult brain. For the abdomen, moreover, the strongest signals are often from air bubbles.

Audible sound behaves the same way. A submerged swimmer hears no poolside chatter because of the differences in density and compressibility of air and water. Practically no sound can cross the surface between them— all that strikes it from either side is reflected back.

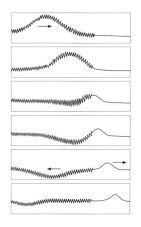

Figure 78. Reflection occurs when a wave moving along a wire coil encounters a segment of different weight or springiness.

TABLE 1

FRACTION OF ULTRASOUND PULSE ENERGY
REFLECTED AT BIOLOGICAL INTERFACES

Interface	Fraction of ultrasound energy reflected
Muscle-fat	1/100
Muscle-bone	1/4
Muscle-air	999/1000

Most soft tissues other than fat have nearly the same density. Variations in acoustic characteristics among the organs are therefore due primarily to differences in elasticity. The elasticity, in turn, is largely determined by the nature of the material that binds the cells of the tissue together, in particular, the structural protein collagen. Thus, much of the ability to differentiate among organs with ultrasound is attributable to differences in their collagen content. Diseases that alter the nature or amount of the collagen within an organ (e.g., cirrhosis of the liver, and some cancers) may give rise to clinically significant image patterns.

The intensity of an echo coming back from a boundary between two tissues depends not only on the difference in their gross physical properties, but also on the size and flatness of the interface area. The outline of an object with a large, smooth surface may be easily visualized. Conversely, a region that contains inclusions and irregularities only of very small dimensions (relative to the wavelength of sound in the medium) will seem nearly homogeneous to ultrasound, and its image will be largely devoid of structure. Between these two extreme cases are organs, such as the kidneys, pancreas, spleen, and liver, that contain or are made up of subparts of intermediate size. Reflections at such inclusions, somewhat like the weak scattering of ocean waves passing through the pilings of a pier, manifest as tissue image "texture," which may be of diagnostic value. Indeed, one exciting area of new research involves the use of computers to recognize certain textural patterns and other image attributes, and to relate them to the effects of various diseases.

SWEEPING THE BEAM
TO CREATE REAL-TIME IMAGES

Ultrasound came into its own as a powerful, flexible diagnostic tool with the development of B-mode imaging. Like CT, B-mode ultrasound uses spatial variations in brightness on a monitor (hence its name) to display the two-dimensional image of a thin slice of anatomy. This involves sweeping a narrow-diameter, pulsed beam back and forth through the body, and making sense of the echoes. The sweep rate, tens of times per

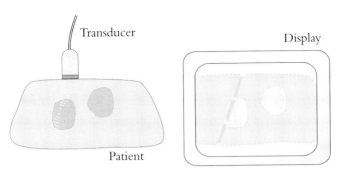

Figure 79. A B-mode image is made up of lines of varying brightness. Each line corresponds to the journey of one pulse of the beam, and a bright point along a line indicates an interface between dissimilar tissues.

second, is slow relative to the rate at which individual pulses are produced, typically 1,000 per second. A modern transducer sweeps the beam electronically, by varying the timing of the emission of the pulses from an array of independent, piezoelectric elements. Then, wherever in the body the beam may be at any instant, and with whatever orientation, the system displays a corresponding line on the monitor (figure 79). The brightness at any point along the line is proportional to the amount of reflection occurring at the corresponding point within the patient, strong reflections and echoes giving rise to bright spots on the line. As the ultrasound beam cuts out a plane through the body, the brightness-modulated lines of display generate a two-dimensional tomographic image. In this manner, up to thirty or so image frames can be produced per second, which is fast enough to distinguish the operation of the heart valves throughout the cardiac cycle.

A modern ultrasound transducer electronically sweeps the beam through management of the timing of the firing of its individual piezoelectric elements (figure 80a). If only a single, small piezoelectric element is excited, the disturbance will radiate out through the nearby soft tissue with a hemispherical wave front (figure 80b). When all the separate elements in a linear array fire simultaneously and with the same amplitude, the separate wavelets will combine to form a flat wave front that propagates outward and parallel to the array (figure 80c). Finally, if adjacent elements are not fired together, but rather are staggered in rapid sequence, the resulting wave front leaves the source at an angle. In figure 80d, element 2 is excited a fraction of a microsecond after element 1 (much less than the duration of an ultrasound pulse), and 3 is delayed by the same amount after 2, and so on; a plane wave comes away from the array at an angle that is determined by the interelement time delay. After all the el-

Earlier B-mode transducers contained a single piezoelectric crystal that would be rocked back and forth, manually or mechanically, as the transducer was slowly slid across the body.

The deeper within the body a reflection occurs, the longer the echo signal takes to arrive back at the transducer and the weaker it will be (because of the natural attenuation of sound passing through matter). "Time gain compensation" makes use of the former phenomenon to offset the latter. It does this by ramping up the gain (volume control) of the receiver during the time that a pulse travels into the body and its echoes are returning, in such a manner as to compensate for signal attenuation along the way. That is, the deeper the tissue interface, the

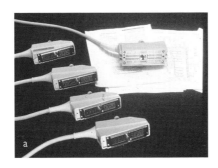
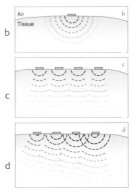

Figure 80. An electronically steered and focused ultrasound beam. (a) The array of small piezoelectric elements of a transducer. (b) Waves produced by the firing of a single element at the skin surface. (c) The flat wave fronts created when all the elements are excited simultaneously. (d) Equally staggered firing of the elements; through control of the delay times among elements, the beam can be swept back and forth and even focused. Figure a courtesy of Acuson, Inc.

weaker an echo will be —but the later it is detected and the more it is amplified. That way the adjusted intensity of the echo from a muscle-bone interface, say, will be nearly independent of the thickness of the overlying muscle layer.

ements in the array have been excited, the computer changes the length of the delay a little, so that the next wave front takes off in a slightly different direction. Generating a sequence of such beams rapidly and systematically one after another causes the ultrasound beam to appear to sweep back and forth. Further refinements yield a narrowly focused, swept beam that is confined to a thin slice of tissue, called the tomographic slice.

MEASURING BLOOD FLOW WITH DOPPLER ULTRASOUND

Have you ever noticed how the whistle of an oncoming train drops suddenly in pitch as the engine charges by? This is an example of the Doppler effect. The same phenomenon can be harnessed to reveal information on the flow of blood.

In a small boat, you bounce up and down more rapidly the faster you move toward oncoming waves (figure 81a). Similarly, when you are moving toward a fixed source of sound, the pitch you hear is higher than what is actually emitted by the source, and the difference increases with your speed. If you are moving away from the source, the apparent frequency is shifted downward instead.

If it is a source of waves that moves, rather than you, the situation is still much the same (figure 81b). A disturbance produced by the source radiates outward as a spherical wave front, centered at the place where the disturbance originated—regardless of the motion of the source. But if the source moves toward you between the generation of consecutive wave crests, then the measured wavelength (the distance between the crests) will be less than what you would find if the source were stationary—and the fre-

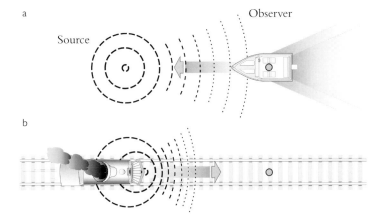

a

Observer

Source

b

Figure 81. The Doppler effect. (a) The apparent frequency of a fixed source of ultrasound increases if the observer moves toward it. (b) The wavelength appears to shorten if the source moves toward the observer.

quency would be correspondingly higher. Once the source passes you by, the detected frequency drops *below* that actually produced by the source. Hence the drop in pitch of the train whistle.

Exactly the same ideas underlie Doppler blood flow measurements. Imagine the red cells in a small volume of blood coursing through a vessel toward an ultrasound beam. Because of their motion, they encounter ultrasound waves of an apparent frequency that is slightly higher than what is actually produced by the transducer. Then, in reflecting this energy, the cells themselves act as an ultrasound "source"—but this new source is moving briskly along the blood vessel, so that the frequency of the echo signal that it re-radiates, and that is detected back at the transducer, is shifted even further upward. The overall effect of the motion of the blood is to raise the frequency of the ultrasound echo that returns to the transducer by an amount proportional to the velocity of the fluid. By measuring the frequency shift, which is technically easy to do, you can calculate the blood velocity directly.

Doppler is commonly employed to detect problems with the flow of blood in the arms and legs, the neck, the breast, and even the eye. Its value used to be limited by an inability to determine the depth of the vessel giving rise to the echo signal. Duplex and color Doppler ultrasound now combine the best of both worlds, matching high-resolution B-mode with Doppler data in ways that reveal the blood flow in a particular region.

The Doppler effect occurs with electromagnetic radiation as well as with sound. It is responsible for the red shift (i.e., shift downward in frequency) of the light reaching us from stars and galaxies that are speeding away from the solar system. Precise measurements of such red shifts are

Just as the speed of a runner can be found from the length and frequency of the strides, likewise the product of the wavelength, λ (in meters), of sound and its frequency, f (cycles per second), gives its velocity, v (meters per second). That is, $\lambda \times f = v$.

of critical importance to astronomers concerned with estimating the distances of the heavenly bodies or with assessing the size and age of the universe. Likewise, as those of us who occasionally cruise the highways a bit too exuberantly well know, police Doppler radar can determine automobile speeds. And it doesn't seem to help much to ask when and how the device was last calibrated.

RISKS FROM DIAGNOSTIC ULTRASOUND

Early in the development of sonar, it was learned that intense bursts of sound energy can kill fish and other small animals. Since that time, the effects of ultrasound on all sorts of living organisms have been studied extensively, and at least three distinct mechanisms have been found that can cause biological harm.

At the high levels of power employed in industry (in the search for faults in metal castings, for example) and in some sonar, ultrasound can cause cavitation (the creation and immediate, violent implosion of microscopic vacuum bubbles) in a fluid. Although cavitation would be destructive of tissues, it hardly ever occurs at the low intensities employed in medical diagnosis.

Medium-power ultrasound does not cause cavitation, but it can raise the local temperature of tissue significantly. Indeed, ultrasound heating is put to good use in physical therapy for various soft tissue and joint ailments. But it is unlikely that heating would be a health concern at the power levels employed in normal imaging.

Finally, ultrasound is capable of exerting shearing and twisting forces on small objects suspended in a fluid. The spinning of intracellular particles in ultrasound fields has been observed, as has induced flow of cellular contents. These findings (together with what some observers believe may be indications of ultrasound-induced incidences of fetal abnormalities and other effects in some test mammals) suggest that there *might* exist processes capable of producing biological damage in humans even at moderate levels of exposure. I am aware of no solid evidence, however, indicating that mechanisms such as these, or others yet unknown, actually do cause harm in humans, even human fetuses, at the ultrasound levels used in diagnostic procedures.

The accumulated clinical experience to date strongly corroborates the safety of ultrasound. More than half of all pregnant women in the United States undergo at least one ultrasound examination during pregnancy, and there have been no clear signs of any adverse effects. Most researchers expect that ongoing long-term follow-up epidemiological studies will support the general belief that ultrasound imaging poses no health risks. Still, as with any other clinical procedure, many physicians would agree that it is prudent to employ ultrasound imaging (especially of the unborn) only if there are good medical reasons to do so. It should be performed only with modern, high-quality equipment, moreover, and by fully trained personnel.

BACK DOWN TO EARTH

With the basics of ultrasound under your belt, you may find it interesting to return briefly to the seismic study of figure 74 and draw some comparisons. The geologist from the U.S. Geological Survey who provided the picture also kindly explained what we're seeing:

Sixty explosive shots and 188 sensors (also called geophones or receivers) were evenly spaced along a 500-meter-long straight line, except along one 108-meter stretch where the extremely steep topography made hole drilling too difficult. Each shot was caused by a one-pound can of ammonium nitrate, buried at a depth of about three meters to couple the explosion energy to the ground. (Some experiments have been very big, involving as much as a megaton in the former Soviet Union.)

Unlike ultrasound pulse generation, where all the elements of a transducer are activated at nearly the same instant with every pulse, geologists get only one try. The shots were set off progressively from one end of the seismic line to the other, with plenty of time in between, so that all the receivers could record the echoes from every blast, yielding a rich and redundant data set. The receivers were tuned to 28 Hz, and the computer implemented a type of time gain compensation. The spacing and energy of the blasts allowed a spatial resolution of about one meter at shallow depths.

As with ultrasound, seismography produces images of interfaces in subsurface materials where the density, compressibility, and speed of sound undergo discontinuous changes. These may occur because of variations in rock types, degree of cementation of the rock, the presence of abundant fractures that decrease sound velocity, the presence of water in pore spaces within the rock, and so on. This kind of information can be extremely useful in prospecting for oil or minerals, or in building large surface or underground structures.

A NORMAL PREGNANCY

CASE STUDY

Six months after marrying, forty-one-year-old Julie MacKinney missed her period two months in a row. She and her new husband, John, were ecstatic when a home urine test proved positive for a pregnancy. Because of

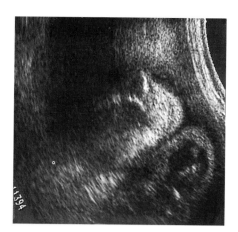

Figure 82. B-mode image of Seth Pearson MacKinney, about seven months after conception. Courtesy of Julie and John MacKinney.

her age, however, this first pregnancy ran higher than average risks, and was watched closely by her obstetrician.

She later underwent an ultrasound study, for several reasons: the image would reveal the number of fetuses (in this case, one), and perhaps the sex, as well. It could help to estimate the time of conception, from the dimensions of the skull and abdomen, for a better prediction of the delivery date. More important, it could confirm the proper placement of the fetus in the uterus (as opposed to within a fallopian tube, for example)—and the absence of a number of other possible fetal abnormalities. Finally, ultrasound could help guide the performance of amniocentesis, to further rule out birth defects.

Ms. MacKinney's ultrasound images revealed the head, arms, and legs of what appeared to be a perfectly formed, healthy fetus. The amniocentesis, performed at the same time, supported this assessment. Figure 82 shows Seth MacKinney in a later image, a few months before his birth, when the features were much more recognizable. We'll update you on all three MacKinneys in the next edition.

8

A Watery Mirror

MAGNETIC RESONANCE
IMAGING (MRI)

"Reflecting in a watery mirror"
T. S. Eliot, *Little Gidding*

Magnetic resonance imaging (MRI) is among the more promising, and certainly the most celebrated, of the imaging modalities. It seems capable of doing nearly everything that computed tomography does, and much more. Like CT, it provides high-quality, thin-slice anatomical pictures, as with figure 14b, but the contrast between the organs and other soft tissues may be a good deal better. Whereas CT directly obtains only transverse images, moreover, MRI can produce equally good tissue slices at any orientation, as in figure 14c, and superb three-dimensional images, figure 13b. Like nuclear medicine, MRI can also reveal valuable information on the metabolic and physiological status of soft tissues. Finally, MRI carries out all its good deeds with no radiation risk to the patient—there are no X rays and, unlike nuclear medicine, MRI involves only stable, nonradioactive nuclei and a variety of magnetic fields.

A BRIEF HISTORY OF MAGNETISM

The magnetic field is one of the indispensables of modern life. It plays essential roles in generating electricity, powering electric motors, recalling pictures from videotape or displaying them on TV screens, storing computer files, even pumping those wretched sounds out of your teenager's stereo speakers. And, in one of its most glamorous roles, magnetism is at the heart of MRI. But what exactly is magnetism, and what does it do that makes it so important? It's hard to describe it outright, so let's go back to the beginning.

The discovery of magnetism was intimately tied to the early use of iron. As long ago as 4000 B.C., the Egyptians and Mesopotamians fashioned ornaments out of small amounts of iron from fallen meteorites. But although they may have recognized the metal's superiority over copper and bronze in tools and weapons, they had no way to produce significant amounts of it from iron ore. The necessary smelting technology was not developed until about 1500 B.C., by the Hittites in what is now Turkey. Within only a few more centuries, though, the Iron Age was in full swing throughout the Middle East and southeastern Europe, and spreading rapidly.

At some point(s) (estimates vary from 2500 B.C. in China to 800 B.C. in Greece), it was noticed that a certain gray-black, metallic mineral is naturally magnetic. Pieces of the iron ore magnetite (named for the Greek province of Magnesia, where it was mined) cling to unmagnetized iron. Moreover, an iron needle brought into contact with this sort of natural magnet may itself become a magnet and even persist in that condition. Such a magnetizable material is said to be ferromagnetic.

This phenomenon was doubtless viewed as no more than an amusing diversion until some clever soul found the perfect application: a magnetized needle or a piece of magnetite, if suspended by a thread or supported by a cork on water, will twist about and end up aligning north-south. The oldest written reference to compasses comes to us from twelfth-century England; indeed, the common term for magnetite, *lodestone*, derives from the Middle English for "stone that leads." But by then, compasses may well have already been aiding navigation for many hundreds of years.

A major advance in the understanding of magnetism came in 1820 with the discovery, by a Dane named Hans Christian Ørsted, that a wire carrying an electric current causes a compass needle to deflect. A current-carrying wire bent into a few loops, moreover, causes a compass to align perpendicular to the plane of the loops (figure 83). These findings demonstrated two wonderfully mysterious facts of life: first, moving charges, such as electrons flowing along a wire, create a magnetic field; and second, any small magnet that can move about freely, such as a compass needle, will tend to align along a magnetic field already in existence. As we shall see, both of these separate but linked phenomena are of critical importance in MRI.

This observation led André-Marie Ampère to propose, shortly after Ørsted's discovery, that the magnetic field from a piece of magnetized iron is produced by large numbers of microscopic loops of electric current—an interpretation remarkably close to the modern one. To commemorate this and his other work on electricity and magnetism, the internationally adopted unit of electric current is named the "ampere."

Many and various additional studies of electric and magnetic fields followed, culminating in the 1864 publication by James Clerk Maxwell of one of the great landmarks of modern thought, a comprehensive, unified theory of electromagnetism. Maxwell showed, for the first time, how closely electric and magnetic fields are interrelated, and how they can combine to produce waves of electromagnetic energy, such as radio waves,

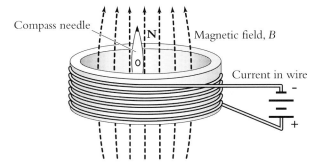

Compass needle — **N** — Magnetic field, *B*

O

Current in wire

Figure 83. Moving charges give rise to a magnetic field. Here, a steady current in a wire, driven by a battery, is producing a field that is fairly uniform at the center of the coil. A compass needle is aligning in the field of this rudimentary electromagnet.

light, and X rays. His work demonstrated that they can propagate through empty space or through matter, and even correctly predicted the speed of light. The crowning achievement in this "classical" description of electromagnetic waves was Albert Einstein's theory of relativity, which revealed, in one of his three great papers of 1905, that electric and magnetic fields are simply two faces of the same entity, the electromagnetic field, seen from different perspectives. All of which brings us to magnetic resonance imaging.

MRI makes essential use of several quite different magnetic fields. One of these, called the principal or external field, is designed to be very strong, homogeneous (uniform) throughout the volume of the patient's body being imaged, and constant over time. The gradient fields, by contrast, are intentionally made to vary in strength from place to place, and are rapidly switched on and off intermittently over time. Still others, the magnetic component of radio frequency fields, oscillate millions of times a second. Different as these are, they do share two important attributes: wherever and whenever you measure it, any magnetic field has both a specific field strength and a definite field orientation. The magnitude and the direction of the field may vary in space and change over time, but at any particular instant and location, both are well defined and unique.

Magnetic field strength is measured in a unit called the tesla (T). The field strength of the Earth itself, viewed as a huge bar magnet, is about 0.00005 T. (Its precise value and direction depend on where you are.) The field strength at the surface of the little magnet that holds your favorite finger painting to the refrigerator door is 0.1 T or so; the magnet may be small, but it is far from weak. MRI is commonly carried out with the principal field in the 0.1 T to 1.5 T range. This is a strong field, by any measure, and it must be stable over time and uniform, to within a few parts per million, over a volume large enough to accommodate a significant part of a patient's body. The technology needed to produce such a field does not come from the local hardware store, nor is it cheap.

As noted in appendix A, gamma and X rays are the most energetic form of electromagnetic radiation, and have the highest frequencies and shortest wavelengths. Ultraviolet is next, followed by visible light—violet and blue down through green, yellow, and red. Below the visible-light range come infrared, microwave, radio frequency (r.f.), and low-frequency radiation.

Something that has both magnitude and direction, such as a magnetic field, is known mathematically as a *vector*. Other examples of vectors include the velocity and acceleration of a moving object and, as we shall soon see, the net magnetization of a collection of protons. The temperature at a specific point, by contrast, has magnitude only, and is called a *scalar*.

The tesla, incidentally, is named after Nikola Tesla, who was born in Croatia of Serbian parents in 1856 and emigrated to America twenty-eight years later. A dreamer and a man of remarkable and far-ranging genius, Tesla invented (along with much else) major elements of the technology that is used, even now, in generating and harnessing electricity. He and George Westinghouse, who bought a number of Tesla's 700 patents, car-ried on an extended battle with Thomas Edison regarding the merits of al-ternating current (AC) versus direct current (DC) power. It was Tesla who got it right.

This brief history would be incomplete without noting that the Earth's own magnetic field tells a long and complex story. Beneath our planet's surface and rock mantle lie an outer core of molten iron and other metals and a solid inner core. Earth's magnetic field is produced by electric cur-rents associated with the rotation and flow of the core materials, which act as a giant fluid dynamo. Shearing and twisting instabilities in this flow have caused variations in the geomagnetic field over the aeons, including even pole reversals, in which the magnetic north pole flops over and ends up near where the south pole had been. This happened most recently about three quarters of a million years ago. Much about the sequence of these events has been inferred from study of the alignments of the mag-netic fields frozen into new rock as it solidified from lava.

It is the flipping over of the magnetic poles of something a bit smaller than the Earth, namely a single proton, that underlies the workings of magnetic resonance imaging.

CASE STUDY MRI FOR THE STROKE THAT ELUDED CT

In chapter 5 and about half an hour ago, we left Frank Pulank suffering signs of a serious stroke, even though nothing showed up on CT. But the radiologist was not overly surprised: the fine blood vessels of the affected area may still retain enough of their structural integrity, even after half a day, to keep the radiographic contrast agent from diffusing out of them and into the brain tissues. An MRI study could produce images like those of CT, but would not necessarily be hampered by the same problem.

At the MRI center, Mr. Pulank was examined, and his medical records were checked, to ensure that he did not have a pacemaker or anything magnetizable within his body that might be affected by the strong or rapidly changing magnetic fields of the MRI device. He was positioned on a table that fed through the aperture of the superconducting magnet, which looks much like the "doughnut" of a CT machine, and the imaging procedure seemed much the same, too (figure 84). The most notable differences are the greater thickness of the doughnut and the length of its

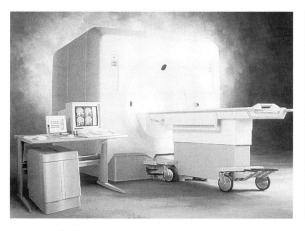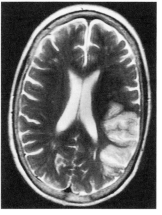

Figure 84 (left). What Mr. Pulank saw: the housing that covers the superconducting magnet of a magnetic resonance imager. Courtesy of General Electric Medical Systems.   Figure 85 (right). Mr. Pulank's T2-weighted image. The lighter area on the right side of the scan is suggestive of an ischemic stroke, in which a blockage prevents blood from reaching a region of brain tissue. Compare with figure 57.

hole, and the frequent, repetitive booming sound, due to mechanical vibrations set up when certain magnetic fields were switched abruptly on and off.

One of the thirty slices taken after administration of MRI contrast material is shown in figure 85. The machine settings are such that normal cerebrospinal fluid shows up as bright, and it can be seen within and surrounding the brain. Healthy brain tissue appears dark. Clearly evident on the right side of the scan is a well-defined irregular area considerably lighter than the rest, consistent with an ischemic stroke. Some swelling of the brain has occurred, and the resulting increased local pressure has compressed the vessels, reducing the rate of blood flow—a phenomenon that an MRI image can sense.

Once MRI had provided the definitive diagnosis, and had cleared up the anomalous CT results in the process, Mr. Pulank was given medication to prevent further clotting, reduce brain swelling, and normalize his blood pressure. The MRI scan suggested that the damage might be reversible. His outcome would depend largely on whether this initial treatment could prevent further short-term damage, and on his body's ability to heal itself over time.

Within a day, Mr. Pulank had recovered some of his memory and speech capabilities. Two days later, he could move his left arm and leg somewhat. He was discharged from the hospital a week after admission. Aided by medication and physical and speech therapy, he has continued to improve—and, to his great joy, Bach is back!

gadolinium, that alter the local magnetic conditions near the water molecules involved in the imaging process.

If a stroke is caught early, and if it is clearly ischemic, it may be possible to dissolve the clot immediately with drugs. The same drugs, however, would exacerbate the situation for a hemorrhagic stroke. Often it is not easy to tell the two cases apart.

MRI USES NMR TO MAP SPIN RELAXATION TIMES OF WATER PROTONS IN TISSUES—GOT IT?

X-ray transmission imaging exploits the partial transparency of the body to high-energy photons. These enter the patient and may, or may not, interact with the electrons of the tissues in their paths. Radiography, fluoroscopy, and CT thus create images of anatomy by detecting variations in electron density (number of electrons per cubic centimeter), primarily, of the different tissues; these, in turn, arise largely from differences in ordinary physical density—such as lungs versus muscle versus bone.

MRI works completely differently! It entails, rather, the mapping out of proton spin relaxation times by performing nuclear magnetic resonance (NMR)—and that, of course, will take some explaining.

Unlike X rays, radio frequency (r.f.) electromagnetic radiation below about 60 MHz will normally pass right through tissues (1 megahertz = 1,000,000 cycles per second). But under highly special conditions, such r.f. energy can be made to interact with atomic nuclei (as opposed to the atomic electrons) by way of the NMR phenomenon.

As it happens, nearly all the nuclei involved in MRI are those of the hydrogen atoms of water molecules within and around cells—and the nucleus of an ordinary hydrogen atom is just a lone proton. Hereafter, we shall refer to these particular hydrogen nuclei as "water protons."

By carrying out NMR voxel by voxel within the body, MRI can map out the amounts of water present or, more precisely, the number of water protons per cubic centimeter or gram of tissue. The greater the number of such hydrogen nuclei in a voxel, as we shall soon see, the stronger its contribution to the NMR signal. But the water proton density (like the electron density sensed by X rays), in turn, depends on tissue type. The resulting proton-density-weighted MRI image may thus be diagnostically useful.

It turns out, however, that the nuclear spin relaxation times of the water protons of tissues are of much greater clinical importance than are proton densities. Chapter 1 gave an example of a relaxation time, but we shall reintroduce this idea here with another analogy, somewhat more in keeping with the spirit of MRI:

Everyone knows that a compass needle naturally points north. There is an irregular, but nonetheless interesting, exception to this rule. Imagine that you are a passenger in a car, holding a rather sluggish compass—one whose case is filled with mineral oil, say. With your fingers, you delicately twist the needle through exactly 180 degrees from its preferred orientation. If you release the needle very carefully, it may stay in this quasi-stable condition for a while, with its "north" end pointing the wrong way, before it eventually flops back into its normal orientation. The average amount of time it takes the needle to be shaken back to its more comfortable state of lowest energy is called a "relaxation time." The bumpier the ride in the car, in general, the shorter will be that relaxation time. You can make the analogy even better by carrying out this little experiment, in your mind's eye, with a tray covered with many compasses pointing the wrong way. Release them all at the same instant; the relaxation time now refers to how long it takes for an arbitrary fraction (63 percent, say) of these compasses to revert to their lower-energy configurations. Now let's relate this to MRI.

As noted in chapter 1, the nucleus of a hydrogen atom, a single proton, behaves somewhat like a tiny compass needle. So for a tissue situated within an intense external magnetic field, most water protons will naturally point along the field, as you would expect. But under highly special circumstances (to be discussed shortly), a detectable number of them can be made to flop over and align briefly in the "wrong" direction, pointing *against* the field. Some of them will flop back to their preferred orientation right away and others will take longer, but on average, they stay in this quasi-stable, higher-energy state for a period of time called T_1. T_1, like the other important nuclear spin relaxation time, T_2, is determined largely by how strongly the nuclei are affected by their molecular surroundings—in effect, by how bumpy their ride is. (Appendix B discusses T_1 and T_2 in greater detail.)

The relevance of all this is that the values of T_1 and T_2 for a tissue can be clinically very revealing. T_1 and T_2 are strongly influenced by the precise manner in which the water molecules are jostling around and bumping into other molecules within the cells. And those interactions, in turn, are so highly sensitive to the fine-tuning of the physiology of the tissues that MRI can produce images that clearly distinguish among the various organs, often much more effectively than CT can.

In the first step toward medical MRI, the American physician and researcher Raymond Damadian found in 1971 that tissues surgically removed from different organs in rats may have significantly different relaxation times (table 2). Damadian learned, moreover, that tumors in some organs tend to have measurably longer NMR relaxation times than do the corresponding healthy tissues. Soon thereafter, Damadian and Paul Lauterbur separately suggested ways in which the NMR signals coming from different parts of the body could be untangled from one another and utilized in imaging. Damadian completed the first whole-body MRI scanner (named "Indomitable," now on permanent display at the Smithsonian Museum; see figure 86a) in 1977; its first picture is shown in figure 86b. These early efforts, followed by the work of hundreds of others, have led to the development of MRI machines that can now map out spatial variations in T_1 or

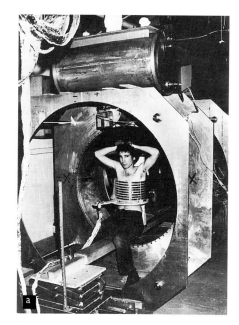
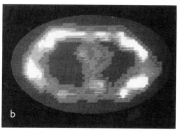
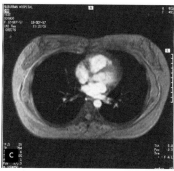

Figure 86. Early days of MRI. (a) The first whole-body MRI scanner, "Indomitable," built by Raymond Damadian in 1977, seen here with slender Lawrence Minkoff in the seat of honor. Damadian himself served as the first guinea pig but was too large for the machine to produce a signal. (b) Indomitable's first image, of Minkoff's chest, took nearly five hours to generate. (c) Roughly the same slice, produced by a modern scanner in seconds. Figures a and b courtesy of the FONAR Corporation; figure c courtesy of Mohsen Gharib, Suburban Hospital, Bethesda, Md.

TABLE 2

VALUES OF T1 AND T2 FOR VARIOUS TISSUE
SAMPLES FRESHLY EXCISED FROM RATS

Material	T_1 (msec.)	T_2 (msec.)	μ(cm^{-1})
normal tissues			
muscle	538	55	0.2128
liver	293	52	0.2167
small intestine	257		
brain	595		0.2079
cancerous tissues			
liver tumor	826	118	
Walker sarcoma	736	100	
water	2680		0.2027

SOURCES: Values for T_1 and T_2 from Raymond Damadian, "Tumor Detection by Nuclear Magnetic Resonance," *Science* 171 (1971): 1151–53; typical values for μ (X-ray attenuation coefficient) from James Mattson and Merrill Simon, *The Pioneers of NMR and Magnetic Resonance in Medicine: The Story of MRI* (Jericho, N.Y.: Bar-Ilan University Press, 1996), 657.

NOTE: Notice how very much larger are the relative differences among T_1 and T_2 values than among the attenuation coefficients—an important factor in the sensitivity of MRI to subtle differences in the properties of soft tissues. $T_2 = T_1$ for non-viscous fluids such as water.

T2 in exquisite detail and with superb soft-tissue contrast (figure 86c). MRI can thus provide useful information not just about anatomy, but also about the physiology of cells, and even about their health.

What do T1 and T2 actually represent, and what do they tell us about the physical properties of a tissue? The biophysics of spin relaxation is a fascinating field, but before exploring it, or addressing the spatial mapping of T1 and T2, we must first talk about nuclear magnetic resonance itself. For now, you need only accept that T1 and T2 are real, measurable times characteristic of certain physical processes that occur on the atomic level—and that they can vary significantly from tissue to tissue because the tissues themselves differ physically.

MRI IS A SPECIALIZED FORM OF NMR

Nuclear magnetic resonance was developed independently in the mid 1940s by Felix Bloch at Stanford University and Edward Purcell at Harvard. The importance of their work was recognized immediately, and the two shared the 1952 Nobel prize in physics for it. NMR quickly proved an invaluable tool for identifying chemical compounds and for studying their molecular structures (and, much later, it even provided a doctoral thesis topic for your author). It also forms the basis for MRI, which burst upon the medical scene in the early 1980s.

NMR involves three fundamental physical phenomena related to magnetic fields. First, as Ørsted discovered nearly two centuries ago, the movement of charged particles gives rise to a magnetic field. A nucleus behaves much like a spinning (hence moving) ball of positive charge; it, too, will therefore generally create a magnetic field, just like the one from a tiny bar magnet or compass needle (figure 87a). As you might suspect from the symmetry of the situation, the direction of a nucleus's magnetic field is closely associated with that of its spin axis: curl your right hand around the nucleus of a hydrogen atom, say, in the direction in which it is rotating; then (by convention) your thumb defines "the direction" of the spin, and points out of the proton's north magnetic pole. A standard measure of the strength of the nuclear magnetic field—that is, of the nucleus's own "magnetness"—is called the gyromagnetic ratio, and designated Γ (an uppercase gamma). Each isotope of every element has its own characteristic value of Γ; and the stronger the field generated by a nucleus, the larger its Γ. For the nucleus of a hydrogen atom, in particular, the value of Γ is 42.57, in the appropriate units.

The second, equally important, basic phenomenon: a magnetized body placed in a magnetic field already in existence will experience a torque, or twisting force, and try to align along that field—which is what makes a

Any nucleus with an odd number of protons or of neutrons will produce a magnetic field. In those nuclei with even numbers of both, the protons will pair up pointing in opposite directions, as will the neutrons, and their fields will cancel out. The nuclei of the common isotopes of carbon, oxygen, and calcium, which together account for about 85 percent of body weight, happen to be of the sort that produce no net magnetic fields (i.e., $\Gamma = 0$ for them), so they play no active role in MRI.

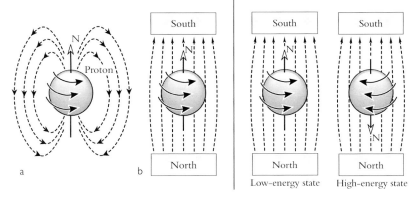

Figure 87 (left). In some respects a proton resembles a tiny bar magnet. (a) It behaves like a spinning positive charge and creates a magnetic field like that of a compass needle. (b) Also like a compass needle, it tends to align in an externally applied magnetic field, such as that produced by the principal magnet of an NMR or MRI device.   Figure 88 (right). When its north pole points toward the south pole of the external magnet, such that the central part of its own magnetic field is aligned parallel to the external field, the proton is in its configuration of lowest energy. But because it is subject to the (sometimes counterintuitive) laws of quantum mechanics, the proton can also remain for long periods of time in the higher-energy spin-orientation state.

compass needle turn. Likewise, a spinning proton placed in a strong external field, such as that of an MRI machine, will have a tendency to settle into the orientation of lowest energy, such that its own north pole points toward the south pole of the external magnet, with the nuclear magnetic field that it itself generates lying parallel to the external field, as in figure 87b.

But a nucleus is subject to the dictates of quantum mechanics rather than the "classical" physical laws that govern the behavior of the objects of our everyday experience, such as compass needles. And under the rule of quantum mechanics, a proton has the option of remaining for an indefinite period of time in a quasi-stable, higher-energy state, spinning in the "wrong" direction, with its nuclear magnetic field pointing *anti*-parallel to the external field (figure 88). So we can speak, hereafter, of the lower- and higher-energy spin-orientation states of a proton in a strong external magnetic field, with its spin lying along or against that field.

Third, suppose you are holding a bar magnet, or the needle of a hefty compass, between the pole faces of a powerful electromagnet. The stronger the bar magnet itself, the harder it will be to twist it over so that it points the wrong way—the greater the effort that is required. Likewise, the energy needed to flip over the compass needle will increase with the strength of the external magnetic field (which we shall represent with the symbol B).

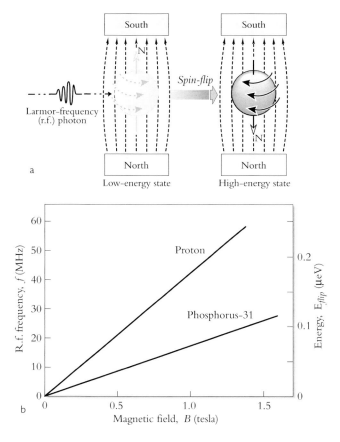

a

Larmor-frequency (r.f.) photon

South · N · South · N

Spin-flip

Low-energy state   High-energy state

North   North

b

Figure 89. The nuclear magnetic resonance phenomenon. (a) NMR involves flipping a nucleus over, in effect, or twisting it through 180 degrees, in a strong external magnetic field, into its higher-energy spin state. The absorption of a photon of the right energy can bring about such a transition. (b) The required energy, E_{flip}, for proton NMR is proportional to the strength of the external magnetic field, B, in tesla (T); see the right-hand axis of the graph. The corresponding photon frequency, called the proton Larmor frequency (left-hand axis of graph), is given by $f = 42.57 \times B$, where the frequency, f, is expressed in megahertz (MHz). The second line is that of the nucleus phosphorus-31, of research interest for MRI.

These three observations apply just as well to a nucleus in the strong magnetic field of a magnetic resonance imager. Picture a nucleus spinning happily in its state of lower energy in an external magnetic field of fixed strength B, somewhere between 0.1 T and 1.5 T, say, with its axis of spin and its own magnetic field pointing upward. The trick in NMR is somehow to grab hold of the nucleus and flip or twist it over through 180 degrees, so that it ends up in the higher-energy state, spinning the opposite way (figure 89a). As you would expect, the amount of energy involved in bringing about this transition, E_{flip}, depends on two factors:

E_{flip} is directly proportional to the magnitude of the nucleus's own inherent magnetic field, as gauged by the gyromagnetic ratio, Γ. That is, $E_{flip} \propto \Gamma$.

The stronger the external magnetic field, the greater the amount of energy needed. Indeed, E_{flip} increases with the external field strength: $E_{flip} \propto B$.

These two ideas can be combined in a single expression, $E_{flip} = \Gamma \times B \times h$, which simply says that the energy required to flip over a nucleus in a magnetic field is proportional both to Γ and to B. The constant of proportionality, h, happens to be a specific, physically significant number, known as Planck's constant, that appears frequently in mathematical descriptions of atomic processes. Since Γ is 42.57 for protons, the energy needed to flip over a water proton in a magnetic field becomes $E_{flip} = 42.57 \times B \times h$. The straight-line dependence of E_{flip} on B for protons is shown in figure 89b. As revealed along the right-hand axis of the graph, E_{flip} is typically in the 0.01 to 0.6 micro-eV (millionth of an electron volt) range. This is a dozen orders of magnitude (a factor of a million million) less than the energies typically involved in X-ray interactions!

We have talked about flipping over protons in a magnetic field, but have not explained how actually to cause these transitions. One process by which a nucleus can be elevated from the lower- to the higher-energy spin state is through the absorption of a photon of the right energy, indicated by the squiggle in figure 89a. Electromagnetic radiation behaves, in some ways, like waves of interwoven electric and magnetic fields propagating through space but, in other ways, it acts as if made up of particles, or localized packets of energy, now called photons. As discussed in appendix A, Einstein demonstrated (in a second extraordinary paper of 1905) that these wave and particle characteristics are related through $E = h \times f$, one of the fundamental ideas of twentieth-century science. E stands for the energy of a (particlelike) photon, f is its (wavelike) frequency, and h is Planck's constant. Equivalently, $f = E / h$. This expression says that the higher the frequency of a wave of electromagnetic radiation, the greater the energy carried by each of the individual photons that comprise it.

Bringing together the main points of the last two paragraphs: a photon that can cause a proton to flip over in an external magnetic field of strength B tesla must be of the exact frequency f (in megahertz, MHz) given by $f = (E_{flip}) / h = (42.57 \times B \times h) / h$, which is to say

$$f = 42.57 \times B.$$

This frequency, at which the nuclear magnetic resonance phenomenon occurs for hydrogen nuclei, is known as the proton Larmor frequency. The relationship between the Larmor frequency for a nucleus and the strength of the external magnetic field, known as the Larmor equation, is illustrated in figure 89b (but this time, refer to the left-hand side of the graph). The Larmor frequency for protons in a 1 tesla field, for example, is 42.57 MHz. In a 0.3 T field, it is 12.77 MHz. Your National Public Radio station, by comparison, operates somewhere in the 88–108 MHz slot allotted to FM broadcasting.

The most obvious method of inducing protons to flip over in a strong magnetic field is to feed them photons of the appropriate Larmor frequency, produced by an ordinary radio transmitter and antenna. And that, in fact, points to a simple method of causing and detecting the NMR phenomenon.

THE WORLD'S SIMPLEST NMR MEASUREMENT

This has all been rather theoretical so far—but what do you actually detect in an NMR (or MRI) study, and how do you carry out the measurements and interpret the results?

Let us design and perform (on paper, at least) the world's simplest NMR experiment (figure 90a). Since the water protons of tissues are the nuclei of concern in clinical MRI, we shall perform our NMR experiment on a sample of water. We begin with a standard radio transmitter that pumps r.f. energy of a single, fairly low frequency (like 1 MHz) into an antenna. We arrange things so that this antenna transmits a beam of r.f. photons through an empty glass tank to a receiver antenna, which is attached to a power meter, and the meter reading is noted.

Next, let's fill the tank with water. Pure water is practically transparent to 1 MHz electromagnetic energy, as it is to light, so the amount of r.f. power reaching the meter does not change appreciably. Then an electromagnet is turned on, and adjusted so that its magnetic field within the water sample is uniform and exactly 1 T in strength. Again, nothing. Is this supposed to be an experiment where something happens, or what?

Now we slowly but steadily increase the frequency of the transmitted r.f. radiation, holding the transmitted power level constant, and plot the detected power as a function of this frequency (figure 90b). The reading of the r.f. power meter remains unchanged up to 42.57 MHz, at which point it dips sharply. That is the indication that NMR is taking place. Here, and only here, some Larmor-frequency photons are being absorbed in the process of exciting water protons into the higher-energy state— NMR is occurring—so less energy reaches the detector antenna. Then, as the transmitter frequency continues sweeping upward, through and beyond the resonance condition, the detected power returns to its previous level. It's like slowly dialing up the frequency of your radio until you suddenly hit your favorite soft rock station. Nothing much happens until the conditions are perfect, but then the signal is just what your weary soul needed.

If the whole experiment is repeated with several different fixed settings of the magnetic field, this same NMR phenomenon recurs (figure 90c)— in each case at the Larmor frequency corresponding to the current value

This experimental approach will work, under ideal conditions, but it isn't how NMR is normally carried out. With a few minor changes in the details, however, it does accurately portray the closely related process of electron paramagnetic resonance (EPR; also known as electron spin resonance, or ESR) in which it is the electrons (not the nuclei) of certain unusual molecules that undergo spin flips. EPR is used widely in biomedical and other research, and is even being explored as the basis for a new form of imaging.

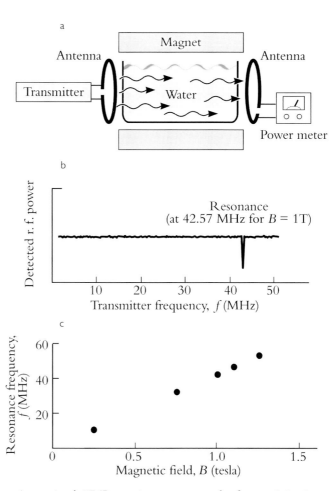

Figure 90. A very simple NMR experiment, on a sample of water sitting in a uniform magnetic field fixed at exactly one tesla. (a) A transmitter generates 1 MHz photons, and a power meter reveals how much photon energy travels all the way through the water sample. (b) The photon frequency is slowly increased; the level of detected r.f. power remains the same, except at the Larmor resonant frequency (42.57 MHz at 1 T), where it dips sharply. (c) The Larmor frequency is proportional to external field strength, in accord with the Larmor equation and figure 89b.

of the field strength, as shown earlier in figure 89b. We have just experimentally demonstrated NMR, the main phenomenon upon which MRI is built!

THE WORLD'S SIMPLEST MRI STUDY—OF A ONE-DIMENSIONAL PATIENT

The above experiment suggests an easy way to map out water proton density (number of water hydrogen nuclei per cubic centimeter of tissue) within a body, or at least throughout the phantom of figure 91a. Our patient consists of a number of thin-walled, pancake-shaped chambers, all

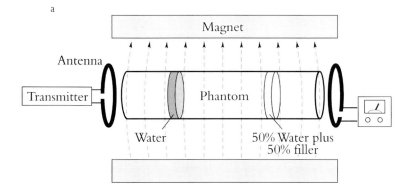

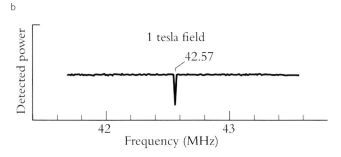

Figure 91. MRI on a cylindrical (quasi-one-dimensional) phantom that is hollow except for a disk-shaped compartment of water one-fourth of the way from its foot, and a disk of water plus Styrofoam one-fourth of the way from its head. (a) NMR with the phantom in a uniform 1 T field. (b) A resonance signal occurs at 42.57 MHz.

but two of which are empty. One non-empty compartment, located one-fourth of the way in from the left, contains pure water. The second, the same distance in from the right, contains a half-and-half mixture of water and inert filler, like Styrofoam, so the average proton density is only half that of water. Our objective here is to determine experimentally the water content of this quasi-one-dimensional patient as a function of position along it. The resulting map of variations in its proton density will be a real MRI image.

With the experimental setup of figure 91a, and with a *uniform* 1 tesla principal magnetic field, the water molecules in the two filled compartments all undergo resonance together at 42.57 MHz (figure 91b), the value we found in figure 90. Not very exciting.

By canting the magnet pole faces somewhat relative to one another, however, we can superimpose a magnetic field gradient on the principal field (figure 92a). The net field is still aligned vertically everywhere (except near its fringes), but its strength now increases from left to right along the phantom. In this example, the field strength happens to be 0.99 T at the

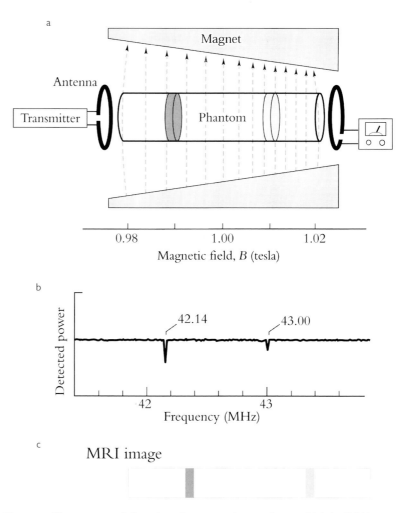

Figure 92. The magnet pole faces have been canted somewhat, and (a) the field is weaker (0.99 T) at the phantom's water compartment to the left than at the one on the right (1.01 T). (b) Now one NMR signal appears at 42.14 MHz (slightly lower than 42.57 MHz found earlier for a 1.00 T field), and another, half as strong, at 43.00 MHz. It is thus possible to relate proton density (from the NMR signal amplitude) to position along the body (from the NMR signal frequency). (c) From this information alone, you can construct a map of the water proton density throughout the phantom—i.e., an MRI image of it.

water chamber to the left, and 1.01 T at the one to the right. When the NMR experiment is performed anew, one resonance signal occurs at 42.14 MHz, and a second, of half the amplitude, appears at 43.00 MHz (figure 92b).

The frequency of an NMR peak (which is easy to measure precisely) indicates, through the Larmor equation, the local magnetic field strength. But field strength increases in a controlled and known manner along the length of the phantom. We have established a way to distinguish the

NMR signals that come from different parts of the body. Not only that, but the amplitude of the NMR signal at any r.f. frequency reflects the number of protons undergoing resonance at the corresponding field strength, hence at the corresponding position along the phantom. Thus measuring NMR signal amplitude as a function of r.f. frequency allows us to determine the proton density as a function of position within the phantom. This is enough data for us to calculate and display a map of water content for our phantom—a true MRI image (figure 92c)! The form of magnetic resonance imaging illustrated here is known as proton-density-weighted MRI.

It is possible to produce a magnetic resonance image of a real, three-dimensional anatomic region by performing NMR experiments point by point throughout it. This involves manipulating several magnetic field gradients and the r.f. radiation so that conditions are right for the NMR phenomenon to occur at one, but only one, place in the body at a time. The magnetic fields are then altered slightly, and the NMR experiment is repeated at another, nearby location, and so on. This approach is much too slow and inefficient to be used in practice, however, and CT-like reconstruction approaches have been devised. These involve the rapid switching on and off of gradient magnetic fields, and the production and detection of numerous carefully sculpted pulses of r.f. energy. A discussion of all this would quickly become quite complicated but, fortunately, the essence of MRI can be understood largely in terms of the simpler picture just sketched around our one-dimensional phantom.

Unlike the situation for computed tomography, one can, in principle, obtain MRI-type information tissue voxel by tissue voxel, by examining each one independently, with no need for reconstruction calculations.

The imaging of proton density is relatively easy to describe, but of much greater clinical importance is the mapping of variations in the tissue water proton spin relaxation times T_1 and T_2. Indeed, the ability of MRI to distinguish among radiologically similar materials, which may look identical with CT, derives ultimately from its ability to reflect spatial changes in these two quantities. We shall return to this issue in a little while.

THE NUTS AND BOLTS OF AN MRI SCANNER

Figure 93 is the block diagram of a generic, off-the-shelf MRI machine. The essential pieces are the principal magnet, the gradient magnets, the radio wave transmission and reception equipment, and the computer.

The component the patient comes into direct contact with is the principal magnet. This must produce a field that is strong (between 0.1 T and 1.5 T), constant over time, and highly uniform throughout a good portion of the body. Commercial MRI magnets are of three very different types: permanent, conventional electromagnetic, and superconducting.

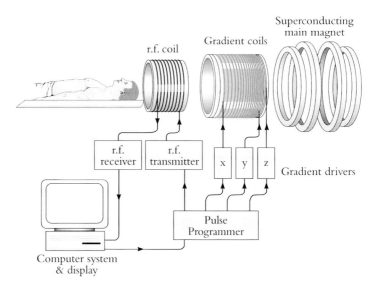

r.f. coil

Gradient coils

Superconducting
main magnet

r.f.
receiver

r.f.
transmitter

x   y   z

Gradient drivers

Computer system
& display

Pulse
Programmer

Figure 93. In an MRI device, the patient is surrounded by the principal magnet, the three gradient coils (energized intermittently by the gradient drivers), and the r.f. coils (radiating pulsed radio frequency power that is produced by the r.f. transmitter). R.f. signals returning from the patient are detected by the r.f. coils and receiver, and then analyzed by the computer.

With a permanent MRI magnet, the vertical main magnetic field is frozen into a hundred or so tons of large blocks of ferromagnetic alloy. Its two poles are situated above and below the patient, which leaves a relatively spacious and nonconfining patient area (because of which the design is said to be "open"), to the relief of patients who suffer from claustrophobia. Permanent magnets can produce only relatively low fields, up to 0.35 T, and some radiologists feel that stronger fields are needed for the highest quality images—but after a decade of sometimes heated debate, it is now generally agreed that permanent magnets are suitable for many routine diagnostic purposes. They are completely passive and require little maintenance; their lower operating costs make them cost-effective in many clinical settings.

An electromagnet, or resistive magnet, such as that of figure 94, looks much like a permanent magnet from the outside, and shares its openness. But its magnetic field, also vertically aligned, is produced totally differently—by driving an electric current through coils of copper wire that lie in the horizontal plane, as in figure 83. This consumes considerable electricity and requires that the heat produced be rapidly removed by coolant water. But an electromagnet can reach 0.6 T, and the improvement in image quality can be noticeable.

The majority of MRI devices produced over the past decade employ a superconducting magnet (figures 84 and 93). A horizontal principal mag-

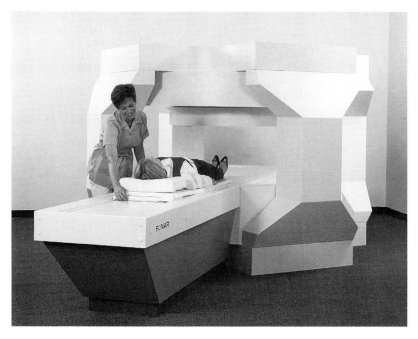

Figure 94. An electromagnet can generate a vertically aligned 0.6 tesla field. (A permanent magnet, which looks much like this, can reach only about 0.35 T, but its pictures are perfectly adequate for many purposes.) The gap between the pole faces is fifty centimeters, enough for a surgeon to operate while watching on the MRI monitor. Courtesy of the FONAR Corporation.

netic field is created by miles of superconducting wire, precisely wound as several coils that ring the patient. Superconducting niobium-titanium metal, for example, conducts electricity with absolutely no resistance; no power input is required to keep the current (hence the magnetic field) going forever, and no heat is generated that has to be removed. But to achieve and maintain the superconducting condition, the entire coil must be immersed in liquid helium (at –270 degrees C, or –450 degrees F, just a few degrees above absolute zero), contained within a doughnut-shaped cryostat (a highly specialized thermos bottle, as in figure 95). The precision manufacture of the magnet / cryostat assembly accounts for a large part of the high cost of a superconducting magnet MRI device. But only superconducting magnets are capable of achieving suitable fields much above 0.6 T, and for some kinds of studies higher magnetic fields are advantageous or necessary. Open superconducting magnets, and magnets that are cooled through electric refrigeration rather than by liquid helium, are being developed and may have a significant influence on what imaging centers purchase in the future.

Also essential to an MRI system are the gradient magnetic fields, like the one illustrated in our one-dimensional imaging example (but produced

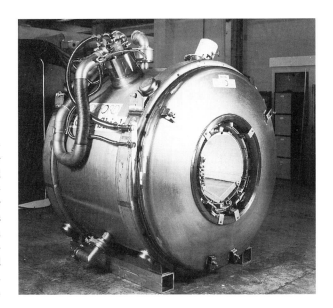

Figure 95. The coils of a superconducting magnet produce a highly uniform horizontal magnetic field up to 1.5 T in strength. The superconducting wires are cooled by liquid helium within a stainless steel thermos vessel to maintain them at an extremely low temperature. Courtesy of Oxford Magnet Technology Limited, Oxford, England.

electrically, rather than by canting the magnet pole faces). Three independent gradient field coils, typically, are intermittently switched on and off throughout a scan, giving rise to muffled, booming sounds.

The radio frequency photons that cause proton spin flips (under the right conditions) are radiated from r.f. coils, which act as antennae. Pulses of r.f. energy are generated and delivered to the coils by the r.f. transmitter. The weak resonance signals coming back from within the patient's body are sensed by the same r.f. coils (or other coils that are placed directly against the patient's body for greater sensitivity). After being amplified by the r.f. receiver, they are sampled, digitized, and entered into the computer.

The precise timing and shaping of the gradient fields and r.f. pulses are under computer control, as are the acquisition and storage of the resonance data. A computer is also required to perform the separate tasks of analyzing the data, carrying out the reconstruction calculations, and processing the resulting images for display.

HAZARDS

MRI does not use gamma or X rays, and so patients and staff are not exposed to any ionizing radiation. The effects on tissues of intense static magnetic fields, switched gradient fields, and pulses of r.f. power have been studied extensively, and none of these appear to pose risks to humans under normal clinical conditions. Studies of the long-term biological effects are under way, but new evidence of problems would be surprising.

In one regard, however, an MRI machine is potentially dangerous and must be treated with respect. Objects of iron and other magnetizable materials can be wrenched about by the principal magnet, and electronic equipment can be affected by the gradient and r.f. fields. Patients or staff who have aneurysm clips, surgical pins, metallic intrauterine devices, shrapnel, artificial heart valves, permanent dentures, cardiac pacemakers, or other metal or electronic items in their bodies should inform the physician or technologist in charge before coming near an MRI device. (Such items often will pose absolutely no problem, but it certainly is advisable to check beforehand.) So, too, should a woman who is pregnant.

Flying car keys, scissors, and screwdrivers can also produce damage. Less critical, of course, but still important is the disruption that an MRI's fields can cause to hearing aids, magnetic credit cards, watches, computer disks, and medical electronic gear.

fMRI, MRA, AND SO FORTH

MRI has earned a reputation in the clinic for providing splendid slice or three-dimensional pictures of anatomy, with additional information on the physiological status of the organs thrown in. But it has also found a number of ways to move far beyond simple, static tissue mapping.

Like PET, functional MRI (fMRI) lights up those parts of the brain that are responding to various stimuli or challenges. Figure 96 shows a front-to-back slice view of the left side of a brain, passing through the eye; "PSM" indicates a region where a difference occurred in MRI images when the subject began tapping the fingers of the right hand. PET can provide analogous information, as was seen in figure 13. The discoveries of such correlations among fMRI, PET blood flow, PET metabolism, and brain activity studies are likely to spur further investigation in all of these areas. As we shall see in chapter 9, other interesting (but low-spatial-resolution) modalities are now being explored for mapping brain function, such as electroencephalography (EEG) and magnetoencephalography (MEG); establishing connections between their results and those of (much higher-resolution) fMRI will be essential for their progress. More immediately, enhancing standard MRI with fMRI can assist in the planning of delicate operations; not only can a neurosurgeon see exactly where a brain tumor is, for example, but she can also assess more fully losses of cognitive, sensory, or motor abilities that might be caused by damage to nearby healthy tissues.

Spin relaxation times of protons are affected by the bulk flow of their water molecules within spatially or temporally varying magnetic fields. As a consequence, MRI can be harnessed to image the blood within the ar-

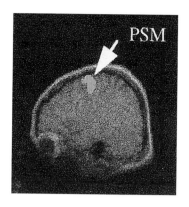

Figure 96. Front-to-back slice through the left side of the brain and left eye. The "PSM" (contralateral primary sensorimotor cortex) arrow indicates one of several areas where a statistically significant difference occurred in the MRI image when the subject began tapping the fingers of the right hand. Courtesy of Venkata S. Mattay, David Weinberger, and Joseph A. Frank, National Institutes of Health.

teries and veins, providing an approach to angiography (called magnetic resonance angiography, or MRA) that is radically different from that of fluoroscopy or DSA (see figure 5c). As with Doppler ultrasound, MRA can assess the rate of blood flow in the vessels, but with much greater resolution and ability to distinguish among them; and it can also display the vascular structure in three dimensions. MRA might provide one roundabout route to breast imaging, for example, since a tumor greatly alters the local vessel architecture. The related technique of diffusion-weighted imaging provides pictures that are particularly effective at picking up early signs of a stroke.

Very fast, gated MRI cardiology techniques can freeze the heart's motions, as with superfast, fifth-generation CT and with MUGA nuclear cardiology. A dedicated cardiac CT device, which can image the heart in a few milliseconds, is highly complex and expensive, however, and generally is cost-effective only in a center that performs a large number of cardiac studies. Nuclear medicine MUGA pictures are relatively easy to make, and they can be very revealing of patterns of blood flow in the coronary arteries, but the resolution is considerably lower than that of CT and MRI. That leaves an important niche that a fairly standard MRI machine with cardiac gating software can fill nicely.

MRI spectroscopy is finding ways to observe certain metabolic processes in tissues by performing NMR on molecules other than water, and on stable isotopes other than hydrogen—in particular, ordinary phosphorus (see figure 89b). Virtually all cellular activities involve the exchange of small amounts of chemical energy, for example, and the standard source of it is the molecule adenosine triphosphate (ATP). MRI spectroscopy can follow the changes in the amount of intact ATP present in a voxel as the molecules donate their energy to worthy biochemical causes, giving up one, two, or three clumps of phosphorus and oxygen atoms in the process. Differences are seen, for example, between muscle

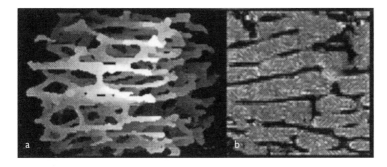

Figure 97. A plane slice and a three-dimensional view of a small cylinder of bone, 0.5 cm across and high, magnified through MRI microscopy. Courtesy of Scott Hwang, Felix Wehrli, and John Williams and the journal *Medical Physics*.

before and after contraction, and between healthy muscles and those that suffer certain biochemical abnormalities.

MRI microscopy is just that—it allows small volumes of tissue imaged by MRI to be blown up considerably in size while still providing adequate image quality. That means that the voxels must be small enough for pixel size to remain acceptable to the eye even after magnification (see figure 47b). In figure 97, a region of trabecular bone (the spongy, as opposed to the smooth, compact, type) one-half centimeter in dimensions is imaged with a pixel size, and resolution, finer than 0.1 mm. When printed out with a laser camera or printer as a six-square-inch image, say, the individual pixels are barely noticeable.

Finally, some researchers are exploring electron paramagnetic resonance (EPR) imaging, which performs magnetic resonance on the electrons (not the nuclei) of unusual molecules known as free radicals. (A radical has one too many or too few electrons than the rules of normal chemistry suggest it should have. Radicals are generated in abundance, albeit fleetingly, when water or tissues are X-irradiated.) EPR was mentioned earlier, in connection with figure 90.

CASE STUDY

MRI DETECTION OF RUPTURED DISK

Four weeks after his automobile crash, described in chapter 4, Bill Herndon underwent a series of MRI scans in search of the cause of the pain and weakness in his lower back and right leg. Of these, longitudinal T1- and T2-weighted studies (i.e., displayed so as to emphasize variations primarily in T1 or T2) of the spine are shown in figure 98, along with a transverse T2. (CT, by comparison, can produce high-quality images only for transverse sections.) Table 3 provides a highly simplified guide to what different materials generally (but not always) look like with T1- and T2-weighted MRI images and CT.

The T1 image provides, as is usually the case, a superb depiction of the anatomy, easily revealing the vertebral bodies and the cushioning disks

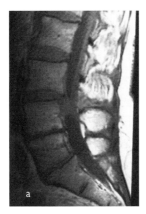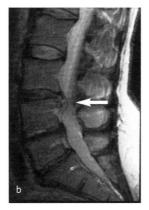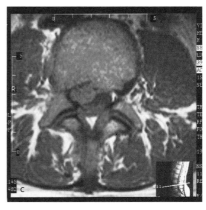

Figure 98. MRI study of a ruptured disk. (a) The sagittal (side-view) T1-weighted image of the spine provides an excellent depiction of its anatomy—in particular, a narrowing of several of the intervertebral disks, indicative of some disk degeneration. (b) The T2 sagittal image picked up tissue abnormalities that the T1 did not highlight. The rupture of one disk, indicated with the arrow, was probably caused by a blow to the spine; a small crack allowed some of the jelly still within the center of the disk to leak out. (c) A transverse T1 image provides precise delineation of the herniation. Courtesy of Bruce Bowen, Washington Imaging Associates, and Health South Diagnostic Centers.

T2 images are particularly sensitive to the accumulation of fluids, and damaged tissues commonly become edematous (swollen with water). Edema, however, is not an issue in the present study.

that separate them (figure 98a). These show no signs of fracture—only a narrowness of several of the disks, which had been picked up earlier on the radiograph. This was suggestive of some disk degeneration, but that alone was unlikely to be the source of Mr. Herndon's problems.

A T2 slice, although not as crisp as a T1, is often much better at detecting abnormalities in tissues (figure 98b). In the T2 longitudinal image, the cerebrospinal fluid, which bathes the brain and spinal cord, appears bright. A normal disk, like the ones higher up in the image, is filled with a kind of aqueous jelly, so its center is also bright. The dark interiors of the lower disks, by contrast, indicate that their jelly has dried out, at least par-

TABLE 3
THE COMMON APPEARANCE OF TISSUES
AND OTHER MATERIALS FOR
T1- AND T2-WEIGHTED MRI AND FOR CT

Material	T1-weighted	T2-weighted	CT
air	dark	dark	darkest
fat	light	light	darker
water	dark	light	intermediate
tumor	dark	light	intermediate
bone	dark	dark	lightest

NOTE: T1-weighted MRI commonly causes materials with short T1 to show up bright, and T2-weighted images are light for long-T2 tissues. With CT, lighter color means denser material.

tially. This often happens with normal aging, though in Mr. Herndon's case, the process may have been exacerbated over time by the physical wear and tear of ranch work. But, again, it was doubtful that this alone precipitated his symptoms.

This image, however, also shows clearly the rupture (herniation) of one disk, indicated with the arrow. A blow to the spine apparently caused that disk to crack open slightly, allowing some of the jelly remaining in it to leak out; figure 98c, a transverse T2 image, provides precise delineation of the herniation. It was the escaped jelly pressing against the nerve that was responsible for the pain and other symptoms. Although the degeneration of the disk probably did not cause the herniation, it did leave the patient more vulnerable to a rupture occurring during the crash. This sort of injury is not common in car accidents, but it does happen.

A week after the MRI scans, Mr. Herndon returned to the operating room to have the damaged disk removed, along with the disk jelly that was pressing on the nerve, and the pain subsided over the next few weeks. He was back on his feet after four days of bed rest, but he was ordered to be extremely gentle with himself for several months.

And oh yes—back to the question of what T1 and T2 actually mean, and why they differ significantly from tissue to tissue: you'll find the answers fascinating, and in appendix B.

9

Epilogue
LOOKING FORWARD

By now, you've probably grown comfortable with many of the basic ideas underlying medical imaging and with the message expressed in the preface and chapter 1: medical images are produced in strikingly different ways, making use of very dissimilar physical processes; as a result, we have a variety of clinical instruments from which to choose in posing and addressing any particular diagnostic question—but we must know how to select the one with the greatest likelihood of providing the correct answer safely and inexpensively. Some of the characteristics of the primary diagnostic tools, and similarities and differences among them—factors that will play significant roles in the selection process—are summarized in table 4.

Several other imaging technologies, some new and some older, may eventually find use in the clinic: thermography, electrocardiography and electroencephalography, magnetoencephalography and magnetocardiography, diaphanography, and tissue impedance imaging.

THERMOGRAPHY

The warmer and bigger something is, the more infrared electromagnetic radiation (heat) it emits. Thermography monitors the heat radiation released naturally through the skin. Irregularities that affect the vascularity

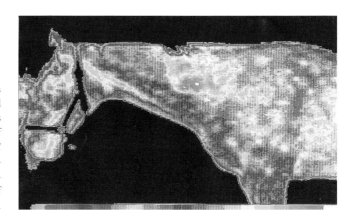

Figure 99. Thermogram of a horse that has recently received an intramuscular injection in its neck. The skin in the region of the injection is about 2 degrees C warmer than elsewhere. Courtesy of Martin Furr, Virginia-Maryland Regional College of Veterinary Medicine.

(the flow of blood) in the outermost quarter centimeter or so of the body's surface, or that influence its temperature in other ways, can be picked up on infrared film or with an infrared video camera. Although it no longer appears suitable for searching for breast tumors, thermography is useful in monitoring inflammatory conditions, such as rheumatic disease, injured muscles, damaged nerve enervation of muscles, burns, and frostbite (figure 99).

ELECTROCARDIOGRAPHY AND ELECTROENCEPHALOGRAPHY

The normal movement of ions within and between active nerve or muscle cells gives rise to weak, transient electric fields. Several methods have been devised to detect and monitor these fields externally, such as electrocardiography (ECG or EKG) and electroencephalography (EEG). In each of these, a few electrodes attached to the skin surface record the faint voltages produced when the heart fires or the brain does whatever it does. At present, it is the time dependencies of the signals that are of clinical value—the shapes or temporal patterns of the voltage pulses—but it is possible that arrays of many electrodes may succeed in generating useful tomographic (i.e., spatial) information as well.

MAGNETOENCEPHALOGRAPHY AND MAGNETOCARDIOGRAPHY

Electric currents within and between the neurons of the brain generate weak, time-varying magnetic fields; from these, magnetoencephalography (MEG) back-calculates the locations and strengths of the neural currents that gave rise to them. The fields are about one billionth as strong as the Earth's, so near-perfect magnetic shielding and a highly sensitive detector are required to map their variations in time and space around the head.

TABLE 4

SOME IMPORTANT ATTRIBUTES OF THE MAJOR IMAGING TECHNOLOGIES

Modality	X-ray film	Fluoroscopy	DSA	CT	Nuclear medicine	Ultrasound	MRI
Probe	high-energy photons (X-ray)	high-energy photons (X-ray)	high-energy photons (X-ray)	high-energy photons (X-ray)	high-energy photons (gamma ray)	high-frequency sound waves	low-energy photons (r.f.)
Source	X-ray tube and generator	X-ray tube and generator	X-ray tube and generator	X-ray tube and generator	radioisotope introduced into body	transmitter, transducer	magnet, r.f. transmitter, and antenna coil
Interaction in body	removed from beam by atomic electrons	removed from beam by atomic electrons	removed from beam by atomic electrons	removed from beam by atomic electrons	(of secondary importance)	reflected at tissue boundaries	NMR of water protons
Detected / imaged by	screen and film	II tube	II tube	array of X-ray detectors	gamma camera	transducer, receiver	antenna coil, r.f. receiver
Tissue characteristics causing contrast	density, thickness, average atomic number	density, thickness, average atomic number	density, thickness, average atomic number	density, thickness, average atomic number	uptake of radiopharmaceutical	elasticity (and density)	water-proton spin relaxation rates
Soft-tissue contrast	low (without contrast agent; but high with)	low (without contrast agent; but high with)	high (uses contrast agent)	high	good to high	good	high
Resolution	very high	good	good	good	low	low	good
Shows anatomy or physiology?	anatomy	anatomy	anatomy	anatomy	physiology	both	both
Cost	lowest	low	medium	high	medium	low	highest

Fortunately, the superconducting quantum interference device (SQUID) fills the latter bill nicely; a SQUID is so responsive that it reportedly can detect the effects on the field of a small magnet caused by someone walking a quarter mile away. MEG has already shown that it may be useful in the study of epilepsy, migraine headaches, and coma. Like PET and functional MRI, moreover, it can also follow the brain's response to stimuli. Magnetocardiography (MCG) is being developed to track the much stronger magnetic field changes that accompany the beating of the heart. Although MEG and MCG are not yet employed widely in medicine, a number of researchers consider them worth vigorous pursuit.

DIAPHANOGRAPHY

Thermography, EEG, EKG, MCG, and MEG all involve extracting information from the electromagnetic radiation that the body itself produces and emits naturally. Diaphanography is a form of transmission imaging that is similar to radiography or fluoroscopy, except that it employs visible-light photons as its probes—as when you shine a bright flashlight through your hand. It is sensitive to the differential attenuation of light (due to absorption and scatter) as it passes through relatively thin volumes of tissues, and records images with either film or a video camera. Transillumination of the breast, for example, can sometimes distinguish between benign and malignant masses, but mammography and ultrasound tend to produce fewer erroneous positive and negative results. It is of some clinical interest, the more so now that researchers are finding ways to prevent light scattered within the tissues from reaching the detector.

TISSUE IMPEDANCE IMAGING

Biological materials contain electrons and ions that can move about, to a greater or lesser extent, in response to an applied electric field. The measure of their responsiveness to externally applied electric pushes and pulls is called their electrical impedance (or their resistance, which is practically the same thing). Tissue impedance imaging assesses the resistance between numerous pairs of electrodes attached to the skin of a region of the body. It does this by applying a low voltage between any two of them and gauging the current produced; it then employs CT-like reconstruction calculations to generate maps of tissue impedance throughout the region. (A major complication is that electric currents do not flow in straight lines.) Like MRI, tissue impedance imaging is sensitive to changes in the water content of tissues; indeed, it is being developed by the military to monitor blood loss from the wounded. Also, since tumors can be much less resistive than normal tissues, it may prove useful in breast imaging.

LOOKING FORWARD

Since we've come this far, why not end with a little speculation on where standard medical imaging may be heading? What might be down the road, just beyond the bend, or perhaps even a bit further on?

First of all, the current image acquisition technologies themselves will improve and broaden in scope. This is immediately evident with MRI, which is spinning off a variety of new tools including functional MRI (fMRI), magnetic resonance angiography (MRA), fast MRI cardiology, MRI spectroscopy, MRI microscopy, imaging with nuclei other than water protons, and possibly even electron paramagnetic resonance (EPR) imaging.

Meanwhile, the speed and resolution of helical and ultra-fast CT continue to increase, and that will doubtless lead to new applications.

In ultrasound (US), we will find better resolution and noise rejection, a larger field of view and possibly higher frame rates, and advances in three-dimensional display. Recently developed US contrast agents (such as foams of microbubbles of air, to be injected into blood vessels) are currently being assessed in the clinic.

Transmission US CT has been demonstrated on relatively homogeneous tissues such as breast, where (as with refraction seismography) variations in sound velocity are measured and processed to create pictures. But reflection US CT, with its multiple echoes, poses severe technical challenges, and progress may be slow.

The solid-state image receptors of digital radiography will get considerably better and perhaps evolve in radically new directions. Similarly, with fluoroscopy, a flat panel consisting of many thousands of tiny, independent, solid-state X-ray sensors (or maybe something else, quite different) may replace the standard image intensifier tube plus camera combination of fluoroscopy. So also for the large sodium iodide crystal and array of photomultiplier tubes of a gamma camera, and for the arrangements of small radiation detectors of some CT and PET machines as well.

It is possible that one or two of the experimental imaging technologies discussed earlier in this chapter may burst successfully onto the clinical scene. High-tech companies are spending a great deal of money to push MRI, CT, combined SPECT / PET, and the other established modalities further—and along the way, they may discover exactly what is needed to bring MEG or tissue impedance or EPR imaging to the fore.

The recent trend in importing ideas, devices, and software from other disciplines will surely grow. NASA and the Defense Advanced Research Projects Agency (DARPA), for example, have developed highly sophisticated imaging techniques to sharpen the eyes of spy satellites, to keep cruise missiles on track, and to search the heavens back to the beginnings of time, and they are now looking for ways to apply their skills to medical diagnosis as well. Similarly, much of the technology that makes modern imaging so vibrant and flexible was produced first by the entertainment and communications industries for games, special effects for films, and so on—and these fields clearly have much more to contribute.

The computer has made its presence increasingly felt in the imaging clinic over the past twenty years, and the excitement has focused primarily on image acquisition and processing. I expect that over the next decade, as we move toward totally digital operation, a good deal of effort will shift over to the faster, higher-volume, and more reliable communication and management of images. Some medical centers have built Picture Archiving and Communications Systems (PACS) to make possible the immediate availability of every image, and all other relevant clinical information, for any patient (see figure 54). A PACS generally has a teleradiology capability, moreover, that allows medical personnel to respond to emergencies from any compatible work station, even at home; to communicate and share images effortlessly with other specialists; and to provide diagnostic expertise in even the remotest geographic areas. PACS got off to a shaky start, largely because they were hyped and then turned out to be somewhat physician-unfriendly. With improvements in the doctor-machine interface, better training provided by vendors and others, and the availability of simpler and more secure mini-PACS that can be upgraded as physicians grow dependent on them, however, it is probable that imaging centers will soon be viewing PACS as indispensable for providing quality health care cost-effectively.

The Internet is already providing a conduit for teleradiology. Opportunities for other applications will expand as the more powerful and versatile Next Generation Internet (NGI) and Internet 2 are established early in the twenty-first century.

Another increasingly important role that computers will play, I think, is in pattern recognition and computer aided diagnosis (CAD), especially with growing access to supercomputers. Computers excel at highly analytic jobs that involve logic and memory, such as playing chess or calculating just about anything. But even the smartest of them have great trouble with the most elementary tasks of everyday life that require intuition, judgment, or common sense, such as interpreting spoken language, or recognizing a face, or distinguishing a liver with an abscess from one that is normal but just looks funny. Still, early results from programs that can search for certain irregularities in mammograms, chest films, ultrasonograms of the liver, and so on, are tantalizing and suggestive of things to come. But it is not yet clear how well, or how fast, computers will progress beyond their current role of offering a "second opinion" on a few special medical conditions.

An important aspect of this effort will be the development of figures of merit for the quality and (not necessarily the same thing) clinical utility of various forms of images. Resolution may be quantified as, say, the minimum separation between two tiny dots or thin lines that can just barely be distinguished from one another, and contrast and noise have their own numerical measures; but although resolution or contrast or noise alone may be critical in certain particular diagnostic tasks, two or all three of them together play major roles in most diagnoses—so it would be extremely helpful if we could find ways to combine these into one or several reliable gauges of image "conspicuity," or overall usefulness. We then could modify the design parameters of an imaging (or pattern recognition, or CAD) system until it reached a maximum in the appropriate figure of diagnostic effectiveness. This is an interesting field of research in which physics and engineering meet psychology on an equal footing, and a great deal of theoretical and developmental work remains to be done in it.

The rapid evolution of basic computer technologies will continue to have a tremendous impact on imaging. One area in which this is immediately obvious is in display. For reasons of weight, size, voltage required, waste heat produced, ruggedness, and—it is hoped—cost, flat panel display (FPD) technology is rushing to replace the traditional cathode-ray tube of the television monitor. Truly three-dimensional viewing, moreover, is now with us. You may have seen stereoscopic drawings and movies, way back when, in which two slightly different perspectives were presented in blue and red lines; you would see those arrows really coming at you when you looked through special glasses with one red and one blue lens (things got totally weird when you reversed them!). Now there are electro-optical "glasses" in which the two lenses themselves can either be transparent, like ordinary glass, or act as separate monitors that display slightly different electronic images for the two eyes, creating the illusion of the perception of depth. They can even switch rapidly back and forth between the two modes, letting you look within two distinct three-dimensional worlds at the same time; for virtual reality applications such as surgical planning or virtual endoscopy, doctors could then interact easily not only with a patient's virtual body, but with one another as well. And with truly holographic display, they wouldn't even need the glasses.

Computers themselves will keep on growing bigger and faster. As of the end of the millennium, the most advanced supercomputers are capable of a trillion, or a million million, arithmetic operations per second. (Your new desktop computer may be able to manage a few hundred million.) Plans are in the works for future computers that will carry out a thousand trillion operations per second, and draw on a million trillion bytes of storage in so doing. What such computational speed and power will do for imaging is hard to predict, but the consequences could be profound.

Beyond designing the ever bigger and faster, some researchers at the cutting edge of computer science are taking the first tentative steps toward building machines that are different in kind, not just in degree. Rather than sending currents of electrons along paths determined by the settings of silicon-based switches, a DNA computer would operate by cutting and joining short strands of DNA in solution; it would consume a billion

The viewing conditions, the training, experience, eyesight, and frame of mind of the interpreting physician, and any available, relevant pieces of clinical information (in addition to the image) that concern the patient can also affect the diagnostic process. It will be important, but even harder, to factor these into figures of merit.

At present, liquid crystal displays (LCD) account for more than 99 percent of all FPDs produced, and are employed in virtually all laptops, but other approaches (such as plasma, field emission, and electroluminescent panel displays) are under development.

times less energy than its solid-state sibling, and take up comparably less space. Another proposed computer would grow as self-assembling clusters of animal or human nerve cells, interfacing with the outside world by way of a semiconductor substrate; it would be literally mind-boggling if such a neuron computer could be made to mimic the structure or function of some of our own neural complexes . . . as a start. Finally, rudimentary quantum computers are being explored that would operate according to the counterintuitive rules of quantum mechanics rather than the normal, if-then Boolean logic of standard computing and of everyday life; they may be able to tackle certain mathematical problems that conventional machines have great trouble with. A success with any of these could radically change computation—and imaging along with it.

Another new area that offers exciting possibilities for medicine is nanotechnology. Microscopic sensors, motors, and other electromechanical devices (which might contain biologic components) are already being manufactured. For medical applications, these could be injected into the bloodstream or bowel, say, and directed to an area of concern, where they might obtain and transmit images, perform chemical tests or biopsies, or even carry out small-scale surgery.

Let us close by posing the ultimate question regarding medical imaging of the near future: how likely is it that anything *totally* new might burst onto the scene over the next few decades? Is another X-ray or CT revolution in the cards? Some if not all of the existing technologies will doubtless evolve and change tremendously, but will we see a completely unanticipated, fundamentally different imaging approach come along?

Medical physicists and biomedical engineers have been hard at work exploring all the physical processes we know of in search of new useful probes—and they don't seem to have stumbled on anything lately that looks particularly promising. This leads some in the field to suggest that what we will see in the imaging clinic of 2025 will be pretty much what we find today, only much, much faster and better. Functional MRI may be fully integrated with PET and MEG, with splendid high-contrast, high-resolution pictures from within arteries being analyzed and diagnosed automatically—but they will still be MRI, PET, and MEG at heart.

Still, you never know.

"Everything that can be invented has been invented."

Charles H. Duell, Commissioner,
U.S. Patent Office, 1899

Protons, Photons, and All That

A BRIEF REVIEW
OF ATOMS AND RADIATION

THE CONSTITUENTS OF MATTER

Everything material is made up of atoms. The air we breathe, the oceans, mountains, cathedrals, water lilies, bumper stickers, computers, butterfly wings, photographic film, and people's hands are composed of atoms. Democritus circulated this idea some 2,400 years ago, but it turned out to be a lot easier to debate than to prove. It was not until the first few years of the twentieth century, in fact, that physicists could provide solid and convincing experimental evidence that atoms were more than just a useful mental construct to help explain the rules of chemistry, as many then believed.

In 1913, Niels Bohr presented the first plausible theory of atomic structure. An atom, Bohr proposed, behaves somewhat like a miniature solar system. Just as relatively light planets orbit a massive sun and are bound to it by the gravitational force, likewise in an atom, relatively light, negatively charged electrons circulate about a much heavier, positively charged nucleus and are held to it by the electric force. But unlike planets, electrons can inhabit only certain discrete, specifically allowed orbitals about their nucleus. Although our current understanding of atoms is based on a highly mathematical and abstract theory known as quantum mechanics, Bohr's much simpler model of the planetary atom provides a picture of an atom that is both easily visualized and largely right, and it will suffice for our purposes.

By the 1930s, physicists had learned that an atomic nucleus is made up of two kinds of heavy particles, positively charged protons and uncharged neutrons. The number of protons in the nucleus (the atomic number) determines the element type of the atom. That, in turn, is responsible for all of the atom's chemical properties and for nearly all of its other physical characteristics as well. The electric charge on an electron is equal in magnitude to that of a proton, but it is of opposite sign. Since the number of electrons of an atom is normally the same as the number of its protons, the atom as a whole is electrically neutral. (The significance of the neutrons is discussed in the chapters on nuclear medicine and magnetic resonance imaging.)

The simplest atom, common hydrogen (represented by the chemical symbol H), consists of a single proton orbited by one electron. The nucleus of an ordinary helium (He) atom contains two protons (and two neutrons), and there are two orbiting electrons. The elements with atomic numbers three through eight are lithium (Li), beryllium (Be), boron (B), carbon (C), nitrogen (N), and oxygen (O). There are about 100 elements, or fundamentally different basic varieties of atoms, and they are listed in your dictionary under *periodic table*.

Atoms rarely exist alone. They nearly always combine to form molecules. A molecule is a collection of two or more atoms held together by electrical forces. Atmospheric oxygen, for example, exists almost entirely in the form of tightly bound pairs of oxygen atoms; molecular oxygen is represented as O_2, where the subscript 2 indicates the number of oxygen atoms in the unit. The two oxygen atoms stick together because each positively charged nucleus exerts an electric pull on every one of sixteen electrons, some of which they share in common. (By analogy, as long as you and your neighbor's fun-loving pit bull are attached to opposite ends of the same arm, the two of you will stay together.) Similarly, a water molecule (H_2O) consists of two hydrogen atoms and one oxygen, all held together by chemical bonds.

Just as chemistry makes sense only in terms of the laws of physics, so also modern biology is largely applied chemistry. Your body contains something like fifty trillion individual, living cells, and each is made up almost entirely of water and four general types of larger molecules: proteins, carbohydrates, fats, and nucleic acids. Within the fourth group is deoxyribonucleic acid (DNA), an extremely long molecule that can store and transmit information, somewhat like a chemical ticker tape. The DNA provides a cell with the information it needs to carry out its appointed biochemical and physiological tasks in a smooth and harmonious fashion.

And it is by damaging a DNA molecule—disrupting its information content (just like randomly altering a letter or two in a ticker tape message)—that X rays may, *extremely* rarely, transform a healthy cell into one that is cancerous.

ELECTROMAGNETIC RADIATION: WAVES

The creation of a medical image normally involves the interaction of some form of radiation with various body tissues, and subsequently with a radiation-sensitive material such as photographic film, a fluorescent screen, or the metal of a radio antenna. But just what is this stuff, "radiation," and how does it actually make contact with matter?

Radiation appears in many guises, and it is commonly defined as energy flowing through space or through some medium like air or water. Perhaps the easiest type of radiation to imagine is sound. Ordinary sound is a mechanical disturbance, waves of compression and rarefaction, propagating through the air. When a drum is struck, the vibrating drum head alternately increases and reduces the pressure in the layer of air directly adjacent to it which, in turn, pushes and pulls on the next layer of air, and so on. The disturbance radiates outward, and eventually reaches and causes displacements of your eardrum, activating some specialized, motion-sensitive nerve cells that send impulses to the brain, eventually resulting in the sensation of a sound. Audible sound consists of such oscillations with frequencies ranging, at most, from about 20 to 20,000 cycles per second, and travels through air at about 770 miles per hour (340 meters per second). Medical ultrasound behaves much the same way in fluids and tissues, but is of much higher frequency (millions of cycles per second).

Also critically important in medical imaging, and in all other aspects of our lives, is electromagnetic radiation. The ancients knew of both electricity and magnetism, but were unaware of any connection between these two seemingly disparate phenomena. Things had hardly changed by the time of the American Revolution, but over the next one hundred years experimenters on both sides of the Atlantic (Ben Franklin being one of the preeminent among them) learned a considerable amount about them both. In 1864, the British physicist James Clerk Maxwell combined them theoretically in a way that implied the existence of propagating waves of interacting electric and magnetic fields. Maxwell's wonderful mathematical theory even estimated the velocity of these electromagnetic waves—about 186,000 miles per second or 300,000,000 meters per second, the measured speed of light!

Gamma and X rays, ultraviolet rays, visible light of all colors, infrared energy, and microwaves and radio waves are all forms of electromagnetic

Energy itself can take many forms, and it is hard to define. But you know it when you see it!

An apple about to fall has *potential* energy because of its position in the Earth's gravitational field. As it drops, its potential energy is transformed into *kinetic* energy of motion. When it strikes the ground, some of that kinetic energy is expended in overcoming the *binding* energy that holds its molecules together; the rest provides *heat* energy to the pieces or is radiated away as *sound* energy. Likewise, heat and *light* energy are given off as wood burns, the chemical reactions of which involve the release of *chemical* energy. And so on.

Energy is a useful construct for one and only one reason: it can be quantified; and if you know how to do the bookkeeping correctly (which may not be so obvious), you always find that the numerical value of the total energy of a whole system does not change during any kind of event or process. Energy is conserved. This mysterious fact of life is one of the most powerful ideas that physicists can draw on in trying to understand and explain how nature works.

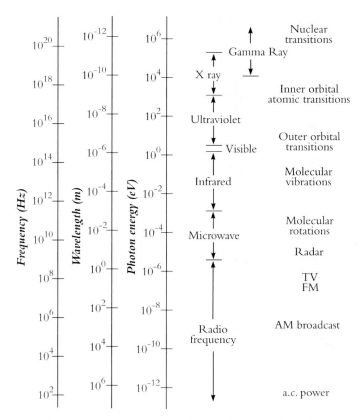

Figure 100. The electromagnetic spectrum. X rays, ultraviolet, light of the various colors, infrared, microwaves, and radio waves differ in wavelength and frequency. Einstein found that the energy of a (particlelike) photon is proportional to the (wavelike) frequency of the associated electromagnetic wave. m = meter; Hz = hertz (cycle per second); eV = an electron volt (unit of energy).

radiation. As with the various notes from a cello, they differ in their frequency and wavelength, as may be seen in figure 100, but in other respects they are inherently very much alike. How the radiation is produced, the mechanisms by which it interacts with matter, and the energy it conveys all *do* depend on the frequency and wavelength. But the essential physical nature of the radiation itself is common to all forms of it and, in many ways, it was described beautifully by Maxwell.

One interesting prediction of the Maxwell theory is that whenever a moving charged particle undergoes a rapid change of speed or direction, a portion of its energy of motion is transformed into electromagnetic radiation. A radio station's antenna emits radio waves, for example, when electrons are driven abruptly back and forth in it by the transmitter. Likewise, so-called bremsstrahlung (German for "braking radiation," as in hitting the brakes of your Harley) X rays are produced when high-velocity electrons slam violently to a halt in the anode of an X-ray tube.

This is the primary mechanism by which standard X-ray systems generate beams for imaging.

ELECTROMAGNETIC RADIATION—PHOTONS

Around the turn of the century, several difficulties with Maxwell's "classical" wave theory surfaced. Experiments showed that light can eject electrons from the surfaces of some unusual (photosensitive) metals. But calculations based on Maxwell's approach indicated that electromagnetic waves should not be able to make this happen. By analogy, even an extremely large ocean wave will not fling a swimmer out of the water and back onto the pier. So what force or substance kicks the electrons out of metal when it is illuminated?

In 1905, the same year he published his first paper on relativity, Einstein proposed that light flows through space in the form of minute, highly concentrated bundles of electromagnetic energy, tightly localized in space. Such localized "quanta" or "photons," unlike Maxwell's spread-out waves, *could* collide with electrons and dislodge them from atoms, and from metal surfaces. Einstein showed, moreover, that although they are alike in some ways, an X-ray photon carries thousands or millions of times more energy than does a much lower-frequency, longer-wavelength photon of visible light. The energy, E, of a particlelike (quantum mechanical) photon, he argued, is proportional to the frequency, f, of the associated Maxwellian (classical) wave:

$$E = h \times f$$

where h, known as Planck's constant, is a physically meaningful numerical constant, and one of the fundamental building blocks of modern physics. Einstein later considered this idea to be among his most revolutionary contributions to physics, and for it he received the Nobel Prize in 1921.

One final but important point about photons: they can be both absorbed and created by atoms and molecules. Imagine a rocket orbiting the sun. We could boost it into a higher, and higher-energy, orbit by turning on its booster engines briefly, thereby imparting energy to it (figure 101a). Likewise, we can excite an atomic electron from its current orbital into a higher-energy orbital with, for example, an incident (incoming) photon providing the necessary additional energy. The photon may collide with the electron and, in the process, knock it into the higher orbital (figure 101b), or perhaps even out of the atom altogether. Either way, an atomic electron will soon drop down into the (just vacated) lower orbital, converting the energy released in the process into a newly created photon, which heads off somewhere at the speed of light.

Some other physically meaningful numerical constants are c, the speed of light, and pi (π), the ratio of the circumference of a circle to its diameter—regardless of its size.

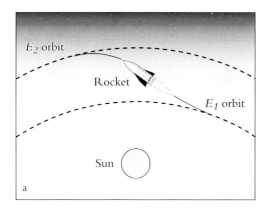 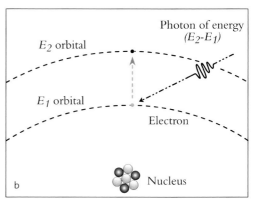

Figure 101. The absorption and emission of photons by matter. (a) You can increase the orbital radius of a rocket circling the sun by firing the engines a bit. The total mechanical energy (kinetic energy of motion plus gravitational potential energy) of the rocket increases from E_1 to E_2. (b) This atom has orbitals that can accommodate electrons with the specific energies E_2 and E_1. A photon of energy $(E_2 - E_1)$ and frequency $f = (E_2 - E_1) / h$ can impart its energy to an atomic electron in the E_1 orbital, elevating it into the higher orbital state.

That, in fact, is the quantum mechanical picture of how you see things. The sun or an electric light bulb produces visible light photons. These travel to, and are absorbed by, the atoms of the objects near you, exciting some electrons into higher-energy orbitals. The excited atoms immediately drop back into their original states, radiating off new light photons in all directions, and some of these enter your eye. There, they initiate very rapid chemical processes in specialized cells (cone and rod nerve cells) in the retina, triggering impulses in the optic nerves which, in turn, stimulate those portions of the brain that give rise to the sensation of a spatial pattern of light. You are unaware of the individuality of the photons because each has but a minuscule impact; countless numbers of them enter your eye every second, though, and you experience only to their collective, averaged-out effect.

More about MRI

T1 AND PROTON
SPIN RELAXATION

An MRI study maps out the way in which one or both of the two clinically significant water proton relaxation times, T1 and T2, vary within a region of the body. But what do T1 and T2 actually represent, and what do they tell us about the physical properties of, say, the brain? The short answer is that T1 and T2 for a tissue are determined largely by the precise nature of the motions of its water molecules—and that, in turn, depends strongly on the type and state of health of the tissue. This all can quickly become rather complicated, however, so to simplify matters, let's begin with something a bit less complex than a brain, namely a glass of water.

Normally, the spins of the hydrogen nuclei of water point randomly in all directions. But suppose you place the glass between the poles of a powerful, vertically aligned electromagnet, and switch the field on abruptly. Each water proton, which is subject to the sometimes counter-intuitive laws of quantum mechanics, immediately snaps into alignment either *along* or *against* the external field—and during that first brief moment of mass confusion, it happens that almost exactly equal numbers of them will end up in the lower- and higher-energy states. Since the same number of proton spins will come to point up or down, the overall, weak magnetic field that they themselves together produce, their *net magnetization*, will initially be zero.

This start-up situation is unstable and does not last. The population of water protons will settle down, over time, and move toward a more comfortable, steady condition known as *thermal equilibrium*. Thermal equilib-

With ordinary compasses, *all* the needles would swing rapidly into the same lowest-energy orientation. But quantum mechanics doesn't place much stock in common sense, and our protons behave quite differently from compasses.

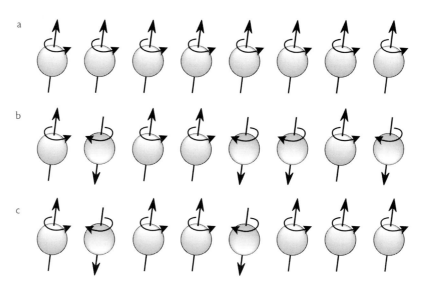

Figure 102. Protons in a strong magnetic field (a) want to align in the orientation of lowest energy, but (b) heavy thermal jostling tends to leave as many spins pointing against the field as along it (entropy maximum). (c) At body temperature, the outcome of this balancing act is a slight excess of protons in the lower-energy state.

rium is established and maintained through the competition of two opposing physical processes. The first is the inclination of each proton to seek a configuration of lowest energy, with its north pole pointing toward the external magnet's south pole (figure 102a). The second is the tendency of a group of vibrating, rotating, and colliding water molecules to jostle one another into a state of greatest disorder, or maximum entropy, with roughly equal numbers of their protons in the two spin orientations (figure 102b). At very low temperatures, the clear-cut winner in the battle between energy and entropy is the former; in laboratory experiments carried out on samples of ice at temperatures near absolute zero, the spins all line up like bowling pins. At very high temperatures, on the other hand, entropy comes out on top—a group of water molecules will be bouncing around and knocking into one another and, at any instant, roughly half the protons find themselves in each spin state. Over time, the individual spins may flip up and down but, once equilibrium is achieved, this overall half-and-half balance remains constant over time.

For water at body temperature, as in MRI, the proton spin system is warm but not hot; it will end up somewhere in between the two extreme-case scenarios just described, in a state that resembles the maximum-entropy situation but which is, in fact, significantly different. A little more than half the water protons find themselves in the lower-energy spin

The same situation resulted from rapidly switching on the external magnetic field, but that was caused by a very different mechanism.

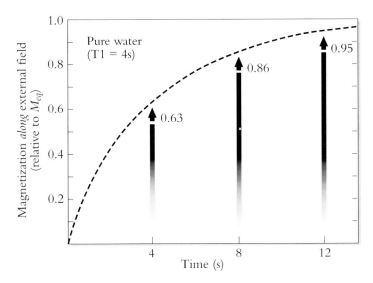

Figure 103. The approach of a disturbed spin system to thermal equilibrium is characterized by the spin relaxation time T1. After a long time, the magnetization reaches its equilibrium value, M_{eq}. Over an interval of duration T1, the system gets only 63 percent of the way there. For pure water at body temperature in a 1.5 T field, T1 is about four seconds. For most normal tissues, T1 is a factor of ten or so shorter than that.

state, with a small but definite excess of protons pointing upward (figure 102c). In a one-tesla magnetic field, for example, the relative *excess* of proton spins pointing north is about three parts per million. That may not seem like much, until we recall that there are seventy billion billion (7×10^{19}) such protons in a cubic millimeter of water. In a volume the size of a typical voxel, there will be an excess of something like a million billion of them in the lower-energy state. This slender margin gives rise to a weak, but measurable, communal magnetic field, the net magnetization of the water protons, which is ultimately responsible for MRI signals.

We have just depicted the *state* of thermal equilibrium of a population of protons at body temperature in a strong magnetic field. It is the *process* itself of moving toward the equilibrium condition through nuclear spin relaxation, however, and the *rate at which this process occurs*, that are of primary interest in MRI. When we switch on the magnetic field, the net magnetization of the protons grows from zero, initially, to its final, equilibrium value, pointing along the external magnetic field—and T1 is the parameter that characterizes how long this process takes (figure 103). T1 is defined, somewhat arbitrarily, as the time required by the system to go a certain part (63 percent) of the way from a configuration of zero net magnetization to equilibrium. As reflected in figure 103, the experimentally measured value of T1 for pure water at body temperature in a 1.5 tesla field

A disturbed spin system returns to equilibrium with a time dependence of $(1 - e^{-t/T1})$. For the particular time $t = T1$, this factor reduces to 0.63.

is several seconds. For most tissues, it is a factor of ten or so shorter than that (see table 2).

Now that you understand what T1 is, and the central role it plays in the overall MRI scheme of things, you are doubtless anxious to take the last few steps, and see what actually determines the length of T1 for a particular material, and how to measure it. Read on!

WHY DO DIFFERENT TISSUES HAVE DIFFERENT VALUES FOR T1 AND T2?

A disturbed system of spins in a strong magnetic field spontaneously evolves toward thermal equilibrium. This must involve proton spin flips—but what is making them happen?

We have seen that one way to induce NMR transitions in a population of spins is to expose it intentionally to Larmor-frequency photons. Analysis of the relevant physics reveals that it is the magnetic (rather than electric) field of a Larmor-frequency photon interacting with the magnetic field of the proton that brings about a spin-flip event. This suggests that *any* magnetic field that happens to be varying at the Larmor frequency could couple with a proton to elevate it from its lower- into its higher-energy state (or, for that matter, to nudge or tickle it down out of the upper into the lower state). That is, if there happen to be naturally occurring magnetic fields in the water sample, some of which are fluctuating at the Larmor frequency, then those fields are perfectly capable of causing a proton flip. Indeed, the stronger the Larmor-frequency component of the naturally fluctuating magnetic field, the more frequently such events take place, and the shorter T1 will be.

Thus we can narrow our focus to the component of those spontaneous magnetic fluctuations (i.e., of the magnetic noise) that happens to be occurring at the Larmor frequency. There are a number of ways that protons can experience such fields. The most important involves the magnetic interaction between the two hydrogen nuclei of the same water molecule. As the molecule bounces around, the spin axis of each proton, and the magnetic field it produces, will tend to remain pointing along or against the strong, constant external magnetic field. But the weak field from one proton will overlap its partner—and the strength of this additional overlap field is determined, at any moment, by the instantaneous relative alignments of the two proton spins, hence on their relative positions in the external field (figure 104). So as the orientation of the water molecule varies, the amount of proton-proton field overlap will change, as well.

When a molecule as a whole is whirling about some axis, each proton feels (in addition to the external magnetic field) the weak field due to its

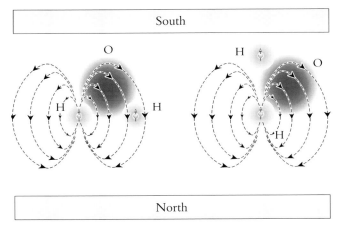

Figure 104. Each hydrogen nucleus of the water molecule aligns either along or against the strong external magnetic field. A proton experiences also the small magnetic field caused by its partner proton. The strength of that inter-proton field depends on the relative orientation of the water molecule in the external field. As the molecule tumbles, the strength of the field produced by one proton and felt by the other varies at the tumble rate.

own partner proton, varying at the molecular rotation frequency. After a short while, the water molecule will collide randomly with another molecule, and begin revolving about a new axis at a different rate. Both of its protons now feel weak fields that oscillate at this new molecular rotational frequency. Such molecular collisions occur again and again, countless times per second. Whenever, during all of this, a water molecule finds itself revolving at the Larmor frequency, then the local magnetic fields at the two protons will also cycle at that rate—and such naturally occurring Larmor-frequency fields can induce proton spin-state transitions.

To summarize: Because of natural proton-proton magnetic interactions, some of which happen to be varying at the Larmor frequency, water protons in a material can undergo spontaneous spin flips. This will allow the proton net magnetization to come to thermal equilibrium, at a rate parameterized by the relaxation time T_1. The rate of equilibration will be fast, and T_1 will be short, if Larmor-frequency magnetic field fluctuations exist in abundance—and the likelihood that water protons will experience such fields is determined largely by the nature of the rotations and other motions of the water molecules themselves.

This explains why different tissues have different values of T_1. In a cell, the motions of the water molecules, and hence the value of T_1, are strongly influenced by how tightly a cell's water molecules interact with various ions or biomolecules in solution, or with the cellular membranes. For water connected firmly to massive proteins, which tumble slowly, the protons would be subjected to proton-overlap fields that vary at the tumble

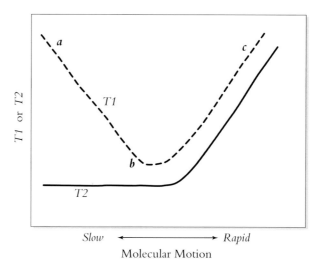

Slow ⟵————————⟶ Rapid

Molecular Motion

Figure 105. T1 depends on the tightness of the bonds between water molecules and the various cellular biomolecules, and on the viscosity of the cellular fluid, among other things. Both affect the rate at which the water molecules move about, and the likelihood that they will experience naturally occurring Larmor-frequency fields. Points a and c refer to conditions in which water protons are experiencing naturally occurring magnetic fields that vary at frequencies much lower and higher than the Larmor frequency, respectively. At point b, protons will undergo spin-state transitions even in the absence of Larmor-frequency photons beamed in from outside, and T1 will be relatively short. As the second curve suggests, low-frequency fields contribute to T2 relaxation.

frequencies (figure 105, point a)—but those tend to be much lower than the proton Larmor frequency, so proton spin relaxation will be slow, and T1 long. A completely free water molecule, on the other hand, is small and light, and will rotate about any axis at a rate much higher than the Larmor frequency, also resulting in a relatively long T1 (figure 105, point c). But water molecules bound to midsized biomolecules, or attached relatively loosely to any sizable biomolecules, may end up rotating at rates close to the Larmor frequency—hence a short T1 (figure 105, point b). The effective, or average, value of T1 for a cell is determined largely by the relative numbers of water molecules encountering the various possible molecular environments. The viscosity of the cellular contents also affects T1, for similar reasons.

The story for T2 is somewhat different, and we shall return to it in the next section.

Numerous normal and abnormal physiologic processes affect the amounts of water residing within cells and experiencing various different molecular environments. These processes can influence the binding of water to the cellular contents, the viscosity of the solution, and other relevant factors, and they are reflected in the measured values of T1 and T2, as in table 2. Put another way: the type and status of health of a tissue determine how much water is in its cells, where it is located, and what is dissolved or suspended in it. That, in turn, has an impact on the motions and local magnetic environments of the individual water molecules—in particular, their ability to rotate at frequencies near the Larmor frequency. And *that* will affect T1 and T2.

This is why spatial variations in the values of T1 and T2 are of such interest: because these water proton spin relaxation times depend on cell type, MRI can distinguish one tissue or organ from another; because they also are affected by the physiological status of a tissue, MRI may even reveal pathological conditions.

It's time now to sit back, stretch, and recognize that you have succeeded in linking the two principal themes of the MRI story—proton NMR for the tissue in a voxel, discussed in chapter 8, and proton spin relaxation there. NMR may be used as a tool to obtain T1 at a specific location within the body—and by repeating this determination point by point throughout a region, you can generate a form of T1-weighted MRI image, in which variations in T1 are predominant. (The approaches actually used in commercial MRI units are quite complex, and much faster, but they provide essentially the same kind of information.) What we have not shown yet, however, is how to use NMR to measure T1 in a voxel. To discuss that, we need to look at NMR from a new perspective.

THE CLASSICAL VIEW OF NMR

NMR has been described, so far, essentially in terms of a single proton that acts in a magnetic field somewhat like a compass needle, but with only two (higher- and lower-energy) possible spin states. There is a completely different view of the phenomenon, called the "classical" description, based on the observation that the net magnetization produced by a population of protons behaves in a magnetic field much like a gyroscope moving about in the Earth's gravitational field.

The classical picture proves helpful in discussing some of the more subtle aspects of NMR—such as why, in practice, NMR and MRI usually involve the application of multiple, brief pulses of r.f., each of which contains a relatively broad band of frequencies, rather than r.f. energy of a single, slowly varying frequency, as in our earlier discussions. The following brief sketch of the classical view, although far from complete, will at least provide something of its flavor.

Newton's First Law asserts that a body tends to remain in its current state of motion, whatever that may be, unless some force (such as a push from the outside, or friction) alters that state. Thus a rocket in deep space,

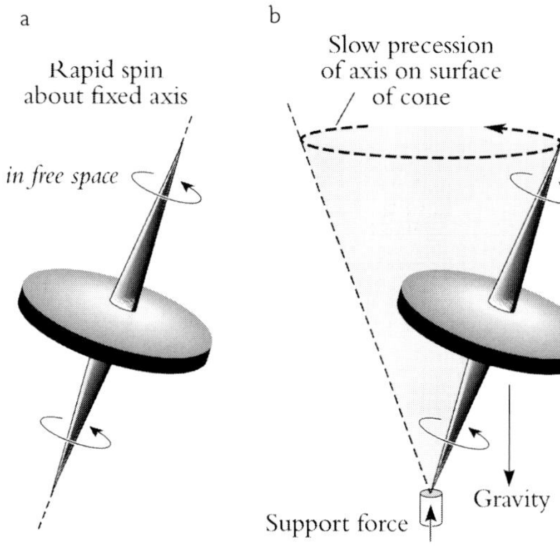

a

Rapid spin
about fixed axis

in free space

b

Slow precession
of axis on surface
of cone

Gravity

Support force

Figure 106. (a) A gyroscope
floating freely in space spins at a
constant rate and about a fixed
axis. (b) But when it rests on one
end in a gravitational field, the
resulting torque will cause it to
precess, wherein its axis of
rotation defines and follows the
surface of a vertical cone.

far from any star or planet that could exert a significant gravitational pull
on it, would proceed indefinitely along a straight line at constant velocity,
as long as it did not fire its engines. Newton's Second Law describes what
happens when an unbalanced force *is* applied to a body. The force of gravity, for example, causes the speed of a falling apple to increase continuously until it hits the ground. Likewise, it is because the Earth lures the
Moon downward, always in a direction nearly perpendicular to its line of
forward motion, that it travels around us in a nearly circular orbit, rather
than flying off on a tangent.

Another kind of motion obeying Newton's laws is rotation. A slowly revolving space station, for example, will just keep on turning about a fixed
axis and at a constant rate (figure 106a). But a child's toy gyroscope spinning on Earth behaves radically differently, since it is subject to two forces
(other than friction): gravity pulls down on it, in effect at the center of the
wheel, and the pedestal supporting the lower end of it pushes upward
(figure 106b). This pair of forces exerts a torque on it, a twisting force, that
is perpendicular to the axis of rotation. The result is a totally new, and perhaps unexpected, kind of motion: the gyroscope undergoes *precession*, a
periodic swinging or wobbling of its axis about the vertical (the direction
of gravity's pull), at a relatively slow, constant rate. The spin-axis defines,
and repeatedly follows, the surface of a vertical cone. It may not be obvious why this should happen—but it can be fully explained in terms of
Newton's Laws. As you might suspect, the stronger the gravitational field,
the faster the precession. A gyroscope on the Moon would precess at one
sixth of its rate here, because the gravitational field is that much weaker
than ours.

A proton acts like a rapidly rotating body, just like the wheel of a gyro-

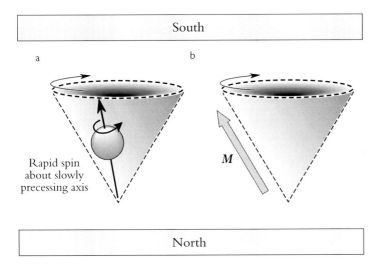

South

a   b

Rapid spin
about slowly   **M**
precessing axis

North

Figure 107. Precession
of net magnetization.
(a) A single proton and
(b) the net magnetization
M of a population of
protons precessing in
a strong, vertically
aligned magnetic field.

scope. It also produces (since it is a moving charge) its own magnetic field,
which can couple with any strong, externally applied magnetic field—and
the interaction between the two fields results in a torque on the proton,
perpendicular to its spin axis. Because of its spin and this torque, the proton's spin axis will precess in the external magnetic field, just as a spinning
gyroscope does in a gravitational field (figure 107a). And, carrying the analogy further, Newton's laws reveal that the frequency, f, of proton precession increases with the strength, B, of the external field as $f = 42.58 \times B$. You
will recognize this as the Larmor equation. The variable f is still called the
proton Larmor frequency, but the interpretation of this classical equation
is quite different from that of the corresponding quantum equation seen
earlier. Before, f represented the frequency of an r.f. photon capable of flipping a proton from the lower- into the higher-energy spin-state in a strong
external magnetic field. Here, it refers to the natural frequency of precession of a proton's spin-axis in that field. Rather miraculously, the two very
different approaches lead to exactly the same Larmor equation. (That's the
kind of thing that makes physics such fun!)

For a population of water protons in a voxel, it is best to consider the
dynamics of the net magnetization, rather than the behavior of any single
proton. We shall represent the net magnetization of a group of protons
with the symbol *M,* written in boldface type to indicate that it is a vector
entity, with both magnitude and direction. *M,* too, will trace out the surface of a cone in an external magnetic field (figure 107b), and the Larmor
equation gives the frequency of its precession.

Let us return to our toy gyroscope, and tack on one additional level of
complexity. We tie a thread to the top of its frame, and start the wheel
spinning. Then, as the toy precesses, we pull very gently on the thread—

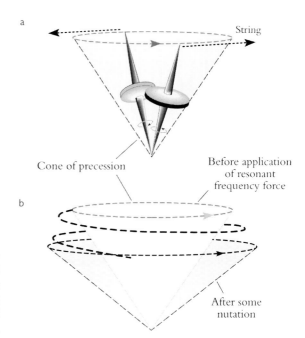

a

String

Cone of precession

Before application
of resonant
frequency force

b

After some
nutation

Figure 108. (a) The nutation of a gyroscope caused by the addition of a second
torque that is perpendicular both to the
axis of rotation and to the torque exerted
by gravity. (b) In nutation, the cone of
precession slowly but steadily opens up.

but always, at any instant, along the direction in which its upper end
happens to be traveling. There are now *two* torques acting on the system—
a strong one due to gravity, and the other caused by the thread—and these
together cause the gyroscope to undergo an even more complicated kind
of motion. In addition to the spin of the wheel about the axis of rotation,
and the precession of that axis about the vertical, the system now undergoes nutation: the conical surface on which the spin axis travels will itself
slowly open up, like a flower unfolding, so that the wheel's axis of rotation
now spirals gently down toward the horizontal (figure 108). Nutation
will occur if, but only if, the direction of the pull on the thread changes at
the rate of precession—that is, this weak, periodic force must be varying
in resonance with the natural precessional motion of the system. If the direction of the force exerted by the thread changed more slowly or rapidly
than the natural precession rate, there would be no nutation.

A radio-frequency coil that produces a weak magnetic field lying perpendicular to the strong, external magnetic field will have the same effect
on the net magnetization of a population of protons that the thread has on
our gyroscope. If the r.f. energy being generated is of a frequency much
above or below the Larmor frequency, M simply continues to precess
about the vertical external field. But if the r.f. radiation happens to be in
resonance with the natural precessional (Larmor) frequency of the system,
it will cause the net magnetization to undergo nutation (figure 109). This
is the classical picture of the NMR phenomenon.

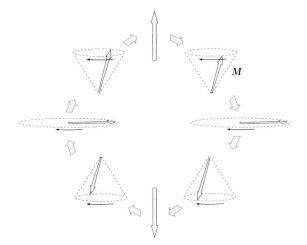

Figure 109. When a coil of wire radiates Larmor frequency power with its magnetic field perpendicular to the strong external field, the net magnetization, M, undergoes nutation.

How can you tell that NMR is actually taking place? The net magnetization might be precessing and nutating like crazy without anybody knowing it. It is easy, though, to make the NMR process reveal itself. Suppose we pump Larmor frequency power into the r.f. coil, exactly long enough for the net magnetization to nutate 90 degrees from along the vertical down into the horizontal plane, and then switch it off (figure 110a). Following application of this "90 degree pulse," M will be precessing at the Larmor frequency in the horizontal plane. Each time M sweeps by, the r.f. coil (now acting as the antenna of an r.f. receiver) will experience the rapidly changing magnetic field it produces (figure 110b). But a changing magnetic field cutting through a coil will induce a voltage in it; that, in fact, is exactly how a generator at an electric power plant works, albeit on a somewhat grander scale. So the appearance of a Larmor frequency signal in the r.f. coil following application of a 90 degree pulse indicates that NMR just took place.

The amplitude of the voltage signal will decay as the proton population re-establishes thermal equilibrium and as it does other interesting things (figure 111). In fact, the time it takes for the signal to drop by 63 percent from its peak value is, in effect, none other than T_2. (Why not T_1? Because of the "other interesting things.")

How might you use 90 degree pulses to measure a spin relaxation time? I'll leave this as something for you to ponder, but I'll give you a big hint: what would you see if you exposed the spin system to a 90 degree pulse, and soon thereafter to a second? What if you did this again, a while later after the system had re-equilibrated, with a somewhat longer interval between the two 90 degree pulses? Enjoy.

Now that we have finally laid all the necessary groundwork, we can

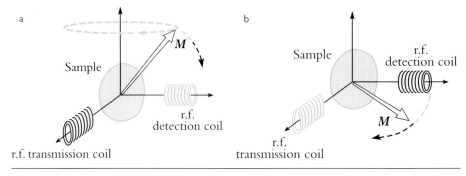

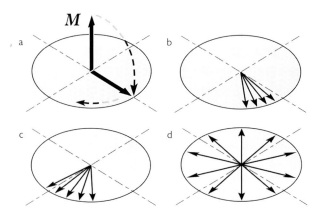

Figure 110 (top). Detecting NMR. (a) Application of a 90 degree pulse causes *M* for the sample to spiral down to the horizontal plane, (b) where it precesses at the Larmor frequency and generates a Larmor frequency signal voltage in the r.f. coil, indicating the occurrence of NMR.   Figure 111 (above). After the net magnetization has been swung down into the horizontal plane by a 90 degree pulse, the Larmor frequency signal detected by the r.f. coil diminishes exponentially over time, with characteristic time T2.

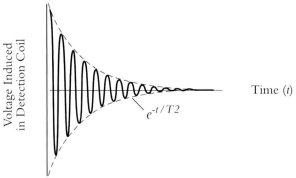

Figure 112. A mechanism that shortens T2 but not T1. Immediately after application of a 90 degree pulse, all protons precess in phase and at *almost* exactly the same rate. The individual protons experience slight but relatively long-lasting differences in local environments, produced by naturally occurring, low-frequency magnetic field fluctuations. They therefore precess at slightly different rates and, after a while, no longer point parallel to one another. The magnetic fields they themselves produce are no longer simply additive, and their net effect, as indicated by the magnitude of *M*, falls to zero with characteristic time T2.

conclude by returning to the second spin relaxation time, T2. Like T1, the time T2 accounts for the thermal equilibration process, so it depends on the Larmor component of magnetic noise. But (unlike T1) it also reflects the slightly dissimilar, relatively "fixed," local magnetic environments in which the water molecules are sitting. Because of local variations in magnetic field that happen to stay put for reasonable periods of time (i.e., the ones corresponding to low-frequency components of the magnetic noise), the individual protons will precess at slightly different rates. This small range in precession rates, and the resultant spreading out in the horizontal plane of the spin axes of the individual protons, are detectable by NMR and MRI, and are incorporated into T2 (figure 112).

Figures 109 and 110 have told a story quite different from that of figures 89 and 90. In particular, whereas the quantum approach suggests that a proton spin-axis can point only up or down, the classical picture has M, and the proton spin-axes, precessing in the horizontal plane. This paradox arises because the spin-up, spin-down quantum perspective and the classical view are both oversimplifications of the real story, which can be presented only with a full quantum mechanical treatment—and it is the two quite different sets of approximations introduced in the simplification processes that lead to the two distinct and easy (but only partially correct) ways of seeing NMR. Fortunately, if you are willing to overlook this awkward little inconsistency, you can use both pictures productively and without getting into trouble.

Suppose that a group of protons happen to be aligned parallel, at some instant, and precessing in phase in the horizontal plane, giving rise to a precessing net magnetization, M, as in figure 110b. Because of the slightly different precessional frequencies of the individual protons, their spin axes will spread out around the cone of precession, and they will lose their phase coherence. The magnitude of the net magnetization will fall as $e^{-t/T2}$, and the signal detected by the r.f. antenna will decay over a time of the order of T2.

Notes

CHAPTER 2

1. H. H. Seliger, "Wilhelm Conrad Röntgen and the Glimmer of Light," *Physics Today*, November 1995, 25.

2. D. D. Patton provides a fascinating and detailed accounting of Roentgen's discovery in "Insights on the Radiologic Centennial—A Historical Perspective, Parts 1–3," *Investigative Radiology* 27 (1992): 408–14; 28 (1993): 51–58, 954–61. Quotation from p. 55.

3. Quoted in A. Pais, *Inward Bound: Of Matter and Forces in the Physical World* (New York: Oxford University Press, 1986), 35.

4. National Cancer Institute and American Cancer Society, Joint Statement on Breast Cancer Screening for Women in Their Forties, March 27, 1997.

CHAPTER 3

1. Quoted in Jerry C. Rosenberg, James G. Schwade, and Vainutis K. Vaitkevicius, "Cancer of the Esophagus," in *Cancer: Principles and Practice of Oncology*, ed. V. T. DeVita, Jr., S. Hellman, and S. A. Rosenberg (Philadelphia: J. B. Lippincott, 1982), 499.

CHAPTER 4

1. Quoted in *Time*, July 15, 1996, 54.

CHAPTER 5

1. A. M. Cormack, "Early Two-Dimensional Reconstruction and Recent Topics Stemming from It," *Science* 209 (1980): 1482–86, quotation on page 1483.

CHAPTER 6

1. Quoted in A. Pais, *Inward Bound: Of Matter and Forces in the Physical World* (New York: Oxford University Press, 1986), 44.

2. Quoted in E. Segrè, *From X-Rays to Quarks: Modern Physicists and Their Discoveries* (New York: W. H. Freeman and Company, 1980), 29.

Suggestions for Further Reading

HISTORY OF RADIOLOGY

Kevles, Bettyann Holtzmann. *Naked to the Bone: Medical Imaging in the Twentieth Century.* New Brunswick, N.J.: Rutgers University Press, 1997.

Kleinfield, Sonny. *A Machine Called Indomitable.* New York: Times Books, 1985.

Mattson, James, and Merrill Simon. *The Pioneers of NMR and Magnetic Resonance in Medicine: The Story of MRI.* Jerico, N.Y.: Bar-Ilan University Press, 1996.

Mould, Richard F. *A Century of X-Rays and Radioactivity in Medicine: With Emphasis on Photographic Records of the Early Years.* Bristol and Philadelphia: Institute of Physics Publishing, 1993.

Webb, Steve. *From the Watching of Shadows: The Origins of Radiological Tomography.* Bristol and New York: Adam Hilger, 1990.

MEDICAL AND HEALTH PHYSICS
(INTERMEDIATE)

Chandra, Ramesh. *Introductory Physics of Nuclear Medicine,* 4th ed. Philadelphia: Lea & Febiger, 1992.

Hendee, William R., and E. Russell Ritenour. *Medical Imaging Physics,* 3d ed. St. Louis, Missouri: Mosby Year Book, 1992.

Shapiro, Jacob. *Radiation Protection: A Guide for Scientists and Physicians,* 3d ed. Cambridge, Mass.: Harvard University Press, 1990.

Smith, Hans-Jørgen, and Frank N. Ranallo. *A Non-Mathematical Approach to Basic MRI.* Madison, Wis.: Medical Physics Publishing Corporation, 1989.

Wolbarst, Anthony Brinton. *Physics of Radiology.* Norwalk, Conn.: Appleton & Lange, 1993. (Highly recommended!)

MEDICAL AND HEALTH PHYSICS (ADVANCED)

Johns, Harold Elford, and John Robert Cunningham. *The Physics of Radiology,* 4th ed. Springfield, Ill.: Charles C. Thomas, 1983.

National Research Council, Committee on the Biological Effects of Ionizing Radiation. *Health Effects of Exposure to Low Levels of Ionizing Radiation: BEIR V.* Washington, D.C.: National Academy Press, 1990.

Webb, Steve, ed. *The Physics of Medical Imaging.* Bristol and Philadelphia: Adam Hilger, 1988.

Webster, John G., ed. *Encyclopedia of Medical Devices and Instrumentation.* New York: John Wiley & Sons, 1988.

COMPUTERS (INTRODUCTORY)

Negroponte, Nicholas. *Being Digital.* New York: Vintage Books, 1996.

White, Ron. *How Computers Work,* 2d ed. Emeryville, Calif.: Ziff-Davis Press, 1995.

COMPUTERS (INTERMEDIATE)

Feynman, Richard P. *Feynman Lectures on Computation.* Reading, Mass.: Addison-Wesley, 1996.

Hennessy, John L., and David A. Patterson. *Computer Organization & Design: The Hardware/Software Interface.* San Francisco: Morgan Kaufmann, 1998.

National Science and Technology Council. *Technologies for the 21st Century: Supplement to the President's FY 1998 Budget.* Washington, D.C.: Executive Office of the President of the United States, 1997.

HISTORY OF PHYSICS

Pais, Abraham. *Inward Bound: Of Matter and Forces in the Physical World.* New York: Oxford University Press, 1986.

Segrè, Emilio. *From X-Rays to Quarks: Modern Physicists and Their Discoveries.* New York: W. H. Freeman, 1980.

Index

Italicized numbers refer to pages with illustrations.

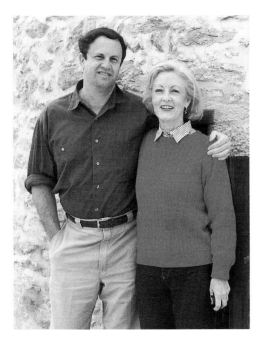

Anthony Brinton Wolbarst, a physicist formerly at Harvard Medical School and the National Cancer Institute, is currently at the U.S. Environmental Protection Agency and an Adjunct Associate Professor at Georgetown University Medical School. Dr. Wolbarst is the author of Symmetry and Quantum Systems: An Introduction to Group Representations *and* Physics of Radiology, *and editor of* Environment in Peril. *His wife, Eleanor Nealon, is Director of the Office of Liaison Activities at NCI.*

Designer: Barbara Jellow

Compositor: Integrated Composition Systems, Inc.

Text: 10/14.5 Cycles

Display: Gill Sans

Printer and Binder: BookCrafters, Inc.